AF333479

A Physician's Guide
to Hypertension

Practical Clinical Guides

Series Editor

Jan I. Drayer, M. D.

G. H. Besselaar Associates
Princeton, New Jersey

Volume 1 **A Physician's Guide to Hypertension** *William B. White*

Additional Volumes in Preparation

A Physician's Guide to Hypertension

William B. White
University of Connecticut School of Medicine
Farmington, Connecticut

MARCEL DEKKER, INC. New York and Basel

Library of Congress Cataloging-in-Publication Data

White, William B.
   A physician's guide to hypertension
   William B. White.
         p.   cm. -- (Practical clinical guides ; v. 1)
      Includes bibliographical references.
      ISBN 0-8247-8231-3 (alk. paper)
      1. Hypertension–Handbooks, manuals, etc.   I. Title.   II. Series.
      [DNLM: 1. Hypertension–diagnosis.   2. Hypertension–therapy.
   WG   340 W582p]
   RC685.H8W48   1990
   616.1'32–dc20
   DNLM/DLC
   for Library of Congress   90-2711
                                                                      CIP

This book is printed on acid-free paper.

Copyright © 1990 MARCEL DEKKER, INC. All Rights Reserved.

Neither this book nor any part may be reproduced or transmitted in any form or by any means, electronic or mechanical, including photocopying, microfilming, and recording, or by any information storage and retrieval system, without permission in writing from the publisher.

MARCEL DEKKER, INC.
270 Madison Avenue, New York, New York 10016

Current printing (last digit):
10 9 8 7 6 5 4 3 2 1

PRINTED IN THE UNITED STATES OF AMERICA

In memory of my mother, Irene Silberman White,
and my father-in-law, Håkon Østvik

Series Introduction

A Physician's Guide to Hypertension by Dr. William B. White is the first in a series of educational guides dedicated to the primary care physician. First-line health care providers need to obtain information related to the patients they see every day in a comprehensive and easy-to-follow fashion. Often, sophisticated textbooks do not provide this kind of information. Therefore, we have started a series of practical clinical guides for the diagnosis and treatment of common diseases. The guides outline what the primary health care provider needs to know to do his or her job best, without going into excessive detail. The guides also include easy-to-comprehend graphs and decision trees to help the physician make sound diagnostic and therapeutic decisions.

Hypertension is one of the most common diseases, and I expect that Dr. White's book will help the primary care physician and other health care providers make decisions based on the etiology and therapy required for the proper management of special groups of hypertensive patients.

Additional clinical guides in the series will follow a similar format and will deal with other common diseases such as asthma, chronic obstructive pulmonary diseases, heart failure, arrhythmias, and Parkinsonism. These guides will help to define which diagnoses can be made and which therapies can be implemented in primary medical care before or after specialty care has been delivered.

Jan I. Drayer, M.D.

Preface

Over the last decade, I have had the opportunity to personally manage over a thousand outpatients and hundreds of inpatients with hypertension in my position as chief of a hypertension and vascular medicine service in a university hospital. Furthermore, our clinical research group in Connecticut has studied several questions in the field of clinical hypertension resulting from my direct observations in practice. Thus, the two disciplines of clinical service and academic inquiry have always been intertwined, and the union of clinical practice and research has been both stimulating and productive for me.

While the largest portion of our ambulatory practice is uncomplicated essential hypertension, I have been most impressed by the effects of other coexisting illnesses on our evaluation process and therapeutic plan. Through my lectures to general medical audiences over the years, I have heard many questions related to issues such as: "Do you treat the home blood pressure or the office blood pressure?" "What is the best therapy for a hypertensive patient with diabetes mellitus?" "If renal insufficiency is present in a hypertensive patient, what is the first test I should order?" Regarding these issues as representative of daily medical practice, this Practical Clinical Guide has been organized to aid in the management of hypertensive patients with these comorbid problems in addition to the important issues of the elderly hypertensive patient, resistant hypertension, and hypertensive emergencies. Thus, the reader will find chapters that address topics such as the management of hypertensive patients with coronary disease, congestive heart failure, diabetes mellitus, "office hypertension," pregnancy, hypercholesterolemia, and so on.

This book is intended for primary care physicians, specifically, general internists and family and general practitioners, as well as physicians-in-training in these respective fields. The primary care physician takes care of the vast majority of patients with hypertension in most countries I have visited. Ambulatory medicine is evolving as a more integral part of the education of our medical residents in both the United States and Europe. I feel it is reasonable that, as our house officers spend more and more time during their residencies in the clinic setting, books about clinical practice will become just as requisite as standard pathophysiology texts.

Most chapters of the book include a case presentation directly from our practice in our hypertension unit. These cases illustrate the problems we see, the evaluation process we consider and/or try, and some of the possible therapeutic regimens we commonly use. A few scientific principles are discussed in each chapter, since clinical practice is based on basic and clinical science. Instead of having a large chapter that attempts to cover all the antihypertensive drugs available these days, drug regimens most appropriate for the individual types of patients discussed in the chapter are highlighted. In this regard, most of the commonly used antihypertensive drugs, alone and in combination, have been discussed.

Writing a single-authored book is relatively time-consuming, and I am not certain I could have completed it without the luxury of being on sabbatical leave, at the University of Bergen, Norway. I am grateful to my department chairman, Dr. James W. Freston, for facilitating my departmental leave from the University of Connecticut Health Center as well as to the several physicians in the Department of Medicine who cared for my patients during my absence. Dr. Per Lund-Johansen, chief of cardiology, Haukeland University Hospital, Bergen, was an exemplary host, incorporating flexibility into our daily schedule that allowed for quite a bit of researching and writing time. I am also appreciative of the excellent work by the medical photography (Fotoavdeling) department at Haukeland Sykehus, which reproduced many of the figures for the book. Finally, the advice and support throughout this year from the editor of the Practical Clinical Guide series, Dr. Jan I. Drayer, and the staff of the publisher, Marcel Dekker, Inc., are greatly appreciated.

William B. White, M. D.

Contents

1

Definitions, Risks, Pathology, and Variability of Hypertension

I. HYPERTENSION—THE CLINICAL CONNECTION TO THE NUMBERS

High blood pressure (BP) is one of the most common chronic adult illnesses managed by primary care physicians. The internist or family physician who diagnoses high blood pressure in a patient and then treats and controls it is actually practicing preventive cardiology for the life of that individual. After all, while the level of the blood pressure is the "symptom" that led to the diagnosis, it is the pathological consequences of high blood pressure that cause excessive morbidity and mortality. The asymptomatic nature of early hypertension can become impressively symptomatic in later stages with the development of devastating vascular and cardiac disorders. This broad spectrum of hypertensive diseases is usually well appreciated by seasoned clinicians who have followed hypertensive patients for one or two decades in their practices.

In some middle-aged and many elderly patients, managing high blood pressure becomes more complicated as other disorders become more prevalent, such as heart and vascular diseases, chronic lung diseases, diabetes mellitus, and sexual dysfunction. At this time, management must be particularly individualized according to the problems that that patient has in addition to hypertension. In some unfortunate hypertensive patients with extensive vascular disease, the problem of management of hypertension may coexist with having to manage severe claudication and rest pain, congestive cardiomyopathies, transient ischemic attacks and/or stroke, renal insufficiency, or perhaps even renal failure. These terminal vascular events are still commonly seen in clinical practice despite much improved antihypertensive treatment. This is due, in part, to the relatively recent (< 10 years) development of some of the available antihypertensive agents and the only very recent recognition of the major impact that risk factors concomitant with hypertension have on the development of cardiovascular diseases.

Therefore, viewing the overall spectrum of hypertensive diseases in your practice provides an impetus for practicing preventive cardiology by proper evaluation and treatment of high blood pressure and enthusiastic counseling and education of your patients. This is an important concept, as we are discussing the treatment of a disease that is, for the most part, entirely asymptomatic and that has met much controversy over the past 10 years regarding its treatment. Throughout this book, hypertension will be observed as a multisystem vascular disease rather than simply an elevated blood pressure from the moment of its time of recognition by the physician.

II. RISKS ASSOCIATED WITH HYPERTENSION

Among the most significant complications of hypertension is acceleration of the atherosclerotic process, which is largely responsible for the increased risk of vascular disease. At present, we recognize that the greatest morbidity and mortality in patients with high blood pressure occur from coronary heart disease. The magnitude of the problem is enormous when considering the 1975 findings of Kannel and Sorlie: simply having three separate clinic blood pressures of over 140/90 mm Hg causes a 37% increase in mortality in men and 53% increase in mortality in women compared to the normotensive population. Furthermore, there does not appear to be a threshold for the increased risk of coronary heart disease in hypertensives; the higher the level of the blood pressure, the greater the risk of a coronary event.

Unfortunately, the results of many large-scale trials of intervention in patients with hypertension have led to a greater controversy than conclusions. Most of the findings from the clinical trials suggest that while morbid events occur at the lower end of the scale of hypertension, the mild hypertensive who lacks other risk factors for vascular disease may derive little benefit from treatment. Thus, the clinician cannot always count on the office blood pressure for finalizing the diagnosis or determining the likely risk of an individual.

Recently, it has become well recognized that the identification and proper treatment of high blood pressure cannot be accomplished without aggressive intervention to prevent or stop patients from smoking. The adverse effects of smoking cigarettes are of great importance in hypertensives, and cessation of smoking may have much more benefit than drug therapy in borderline or even mild hypertension. Cigarette smokers experience an increased incidence of coronary heart disease, peripheral arterial disease, and stroke. Cessation of smoking is associated with reduction in risk for all of the vascular diseases. Results, in 1988, of a large European-based study, the Medical Research Council Working Party (MRC), have shown that while therapy of hypertension induces a reduction in stroke mortality, smoking negates the benefits of the antihypertensive therapy with either thiazide diuretics or beta-adrenergic blocking drugs (Fig. 1.1). Furthermore, there is evidence from the Veterans Administration Cooperative study by Materson et al. in 1988 that hypertensive patients who smoked cigarettes had higher blood pressures and a lesser response to therapy (propranolol) than nonsmokers.

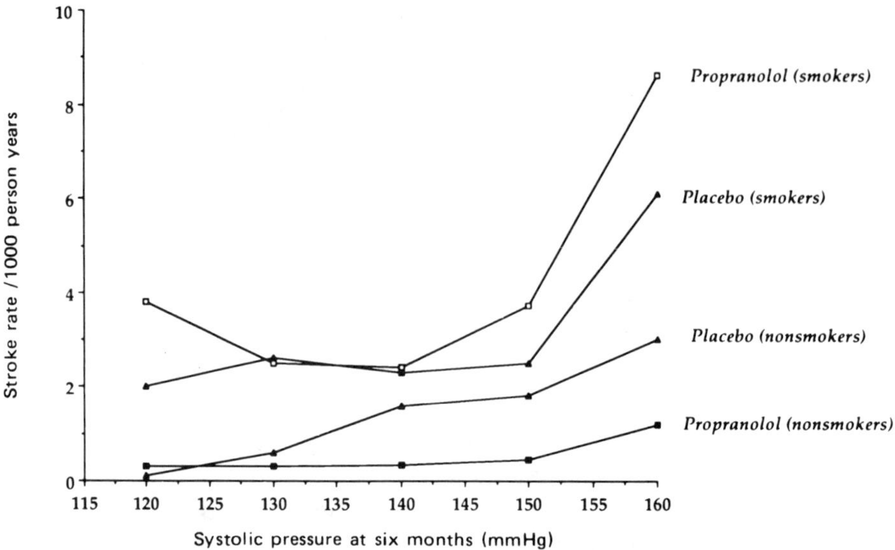

Figure 1.1   Stroke rate per 1000 person-years and systolic blood pressure following 6 months' treatment, according to smoking status. Smoking completely negated the beneficial effects of propranolol therapy. (From Medical Research Council Working Party, *Br J Med* 1988; 296:1565–1570, with permission.)

The most impressive prospective trial to date on the morbidity and mortality associated with hypertension is still the Framingham, Massachusetts study. The twofold rate of mortality of hypertensives compared to normotensives demonstrated in 26 years of observation has basically defined the risk of high blood pressure for the average person in the United States. However, since the inception of the Framingham Heart Study, many Americans have changed their lifestyles and habits (e.g., reducing saturated fat intake, avoiding obesity, increasing the level of dynamic exercise) so that the risk of hypertension as a lone factor for inducing heart and vascular disease may be somewhat different at present.

In different populations in different places in the world, there has been general agreement regarding the morbidity and mortality associated with hypertension. For example, the cardiovascular risks of mild, moderate, or severe hypertension have been found to be fairly similar to the Framingham Study in black and white men in southeast Georgia, according to Deubner et al. (1975); Swedish men born at the beginning of this century, according to Svardssudd and Tibblin (1975); and men and women from the general populus of Wales, United Kingdom, according to Miall and Chin (1982). From the morbidity data in women, it may be true that the definition of hypertension should be adjusted to slightly higher levels in women than in men. Women appear to tolerate hypertension better than men (i.e., it takes higher blood pressures to induce target organ damage in women), but at high levels of BP, the mortality in women is substantial.

It is well known, as reported by Neaton et al. in 1984, that most studies demonstrate that black men and women have higher levels of BP and suffer greater mortality at all levels of BP compared to white men and women. One interesting possible mechanism for the more extreme target organ damage in blacks than whites may be associated with the recent evidence that black hypertensives have a lesser fall in blood pressure during sleep compared to white hypertensives, as reported by Murphy et al. in 1988. This would increase the BP "load" over the 24 hr and could account for the increase in target organ involvement encountered in black hypertensives. This preliminary information is of great interest since it may influence the dosage of antihypertensive medication in patients with elevated nocturnal BP.

III. PATHOLOGICAL CONSEQUENCES OF HYPERTENSION

Two major types of pathophysiological changes occur as a result of chronic pressure overload from hypertension: adaptive and degenerative. Adaptive types of change include both left ventricular and vascular hypertrophy (especially of the small vessels). Degenerative lesions in the heart and arteries eventually occur after many years and can lead to a lethal outcome. The performance of the heart is gradually impaired from a reduction in small vessels supplying the myocardium, increased left ventricular thickness, and coronary atherosclerosis. The main consequence of hypertensive heart disease is the development of ischemic fibrosis, which leads to myocardial infarction and congestive heart failure.

Arterial lesions of medial and intimal hypertrophy are most important in the kidney and the brain. In the kidney, afferent arterioles and some glomeruli become hyalinized, with associated atrophy of the tubules and fibrosis of the interstitium. There is often some impairment in renal function but frank renal failure is rare unless accelerated hypertension occurs. In the brain, small "microaneurysms," called lacunae (dilatation of vessels resembling lakes), develop in the thalamus and may be the cause of a tiny cerebral hemorrhage. Thrombotic strokes arise from arteriosclerosis of larger cerebral vessels or the carotid arteries in the neck.

Most clinicians are aware of the hypertensive changes in small arteries seen in the retina and the classification of Keith, Wagner, and Barker. However, it is often impossible to tell the difference in early changes in the retinal vessels in a hypertensive patient from those of arteriosclerosis (Table 1.1). Nonspecific findings include an increased light reflex, increased tortuosity of the vessels, and arteriovenous nicking. Hypertension, at high levels, will occasionally cause an irregularity of the arteriole with local constriction followed by abnormal dilation. The generalized arteriolar narrowing is a more benign finding and the normal ratio of vein to artery of

Table 1.1   The Retinopathies of Hypertension (and Arteriosclerosis)

Increased light reflex
Narrowed vessel caliber
Arteriovenous crossing defects (associated with arteriosclerosis)
Copper or silver wiring appearance of arterioles
Exudates
Hemorrhages
Papilledema

3:2 is increased. Cotton wool exudates are secondary to ischemia of a retinal arteriole with a microinfarct just proximal to the site of the exudate. The characteristic flame-shaped hemorrhages of hypertensive retinopathy are secondary to a final breakdown of the vessel. Both exudates and hemorrhages are usually pathognomonic of the accelerated or malignant phase of hypertension and pathologically are associated with underlying fibroinoid necrosis. Papilledema is a swelling of the optic disc and is generally thought to be due to a breakdown in autoregulation of capillary flow in the face of high pressure. Papilledema is also nonspecific as any increase in intracranial pressure can cause it to occur.

IV. BLOOD PRESSURE MEASUREMENT AND ITS INHERENT VARIABILITY

Proper blood pressure measurement techniques with either a mercury column or aneroid sphygmomanometer are essential for good clinical practice. Generally, the blood pressure in the office should always be taken in both arms with the patient comfortably seated and then standing with the arm at *heart level*. In many individuals, measuring the BP when the arm is below the level of the heart (while seated or on standing) can artificially raise both systolic and diastolic pressure by 5–20 mm Hg. It is also practically important to take the measurement without a shirt or blouse interfering with venous flow in the arm; even modest venous congestion can elevate the blood pressure.

Miscuffing (using the wrong BP cuff/bladder size) is a common cause of inaccurate BP measurement. In an arm with a midbiceps circumference over 34 cm, a large adult cuff is appropriate, while a small adult cuff is appropriate in a patient with a midbiceps circumference of less than 25 cm. If the cuff size is too small, the blood pressure will be artificially elevated, and if the cuff is too large, the blood pressure will be falsely low.

The risk of target organ involvement and injury is related to the level of office or clinic blood pressure in patients with hypertension. In the last decade though, much has been learned about blood pressure variability in the office versus home or work using portable, ambulatory blood pressure monitors, as reported by Drayer et al. in 1985, Pickering et al. in 1988, and White in 1986. There are individuals whose blood pressure outside of the doctor's office may be markedly less than those in the doctor's office (Fig. 1.2). Furthermore, according to White et al. (1989), there is increasing evidence that patients whose office BP is hypertensive (i.e., $>140/90$ mm Hg) but whose average out-of-the-office blood pressure is normal (i.e., $<135/85$ mm Hg) have no target organ involvement usually associated with hypertension. From the practical standpoint, simple maneuvers can sometimes avoid misdiagnosis. It is important to avoid rushing the patient in the examining room, taking one or two quick blood pressures, making

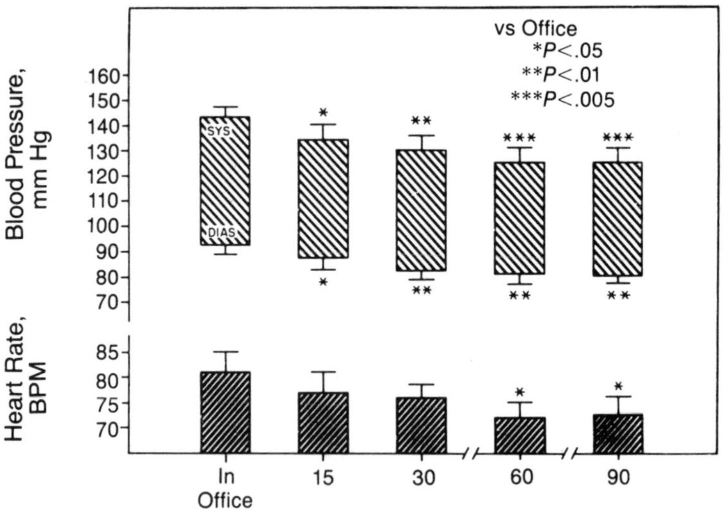

Figure 1.2 Reduction in blood pressure and heart rate in the doctor's office and just after leaving the office in a group of patients with "office" or "white-coat" hypertension. Two-thirds of the patients had average daily blood pressures under 130/80 mm Hg. (From White WB, *Arch Intern Med* 1986; 146:2196–2199, with permission.)

an assessment, and rushing him/her out again. Three or four minutes of conversation is frequently followed by a 10–15 mm Hg reduction in blood pressure in the doctor's presence, according to Mancia et al. (1983).

To demonstrate the variability of blood pressure out of the doctor's office, White and Morganroth in 1989 studied a group of 20 normotensive (office blood pressure averaged 120/80 mm Hg) individuals with automatic ambulatory BP monitoring. The main findings showed that about 10–15% of the awake readings were above a systolic BP of 140 mm Hg or a diastolic of 90 mm Hg (Fig. 1.3). Furthermore, in another group of patients with mild, essential hypertension (again defined by office blood pressures >140/90 mm Hg, averaging 150/99 mm Hg), about 15% have average daily blood pressures under 145/85 mm Hg (Fig. 1.3). Thus, if one took the common arbitrary upper limit for normal BP as 140/90 mm Hg, a patient classified as hypertensive on one occasion may be normal on the next, or vice versa. Thus, it makes practical sense to use multiple measurements over several weeks to months in the office prior to labeling an individual as hypertensive. In most instances, it is wise to take three separate groups of readings (three or four per visit) in the seated position over a period of about 3 months. If a question still exists as to the diagnosis (i.e., one or two readings were in the borderline range), then observation over another 3 months is appropriate. If available, noninvasive ambulatory BP monitoring should be performed in those individuals who have moderate or marked discrepancies (>10–15 mm Hg) between the office and out-of-office (e.g., home or worksite) BPs and in patients who have borderline and variable office BPs.

When considering the diagnosis of hypertension, the seated diastolic BP has commonly been used for a reference value (i.e., >90 mm Hg is a cutoff for the diagnosis). However, some patients with diastolic BPs in the abnormal range have normal systolic BPs in the office (<140 mm Hg) and others with borderline diastolic BPs (85–94 mm Hg) have high systolic BPs (>140 mm Hg). Thus, all of these patients may form different groups, as has been noted

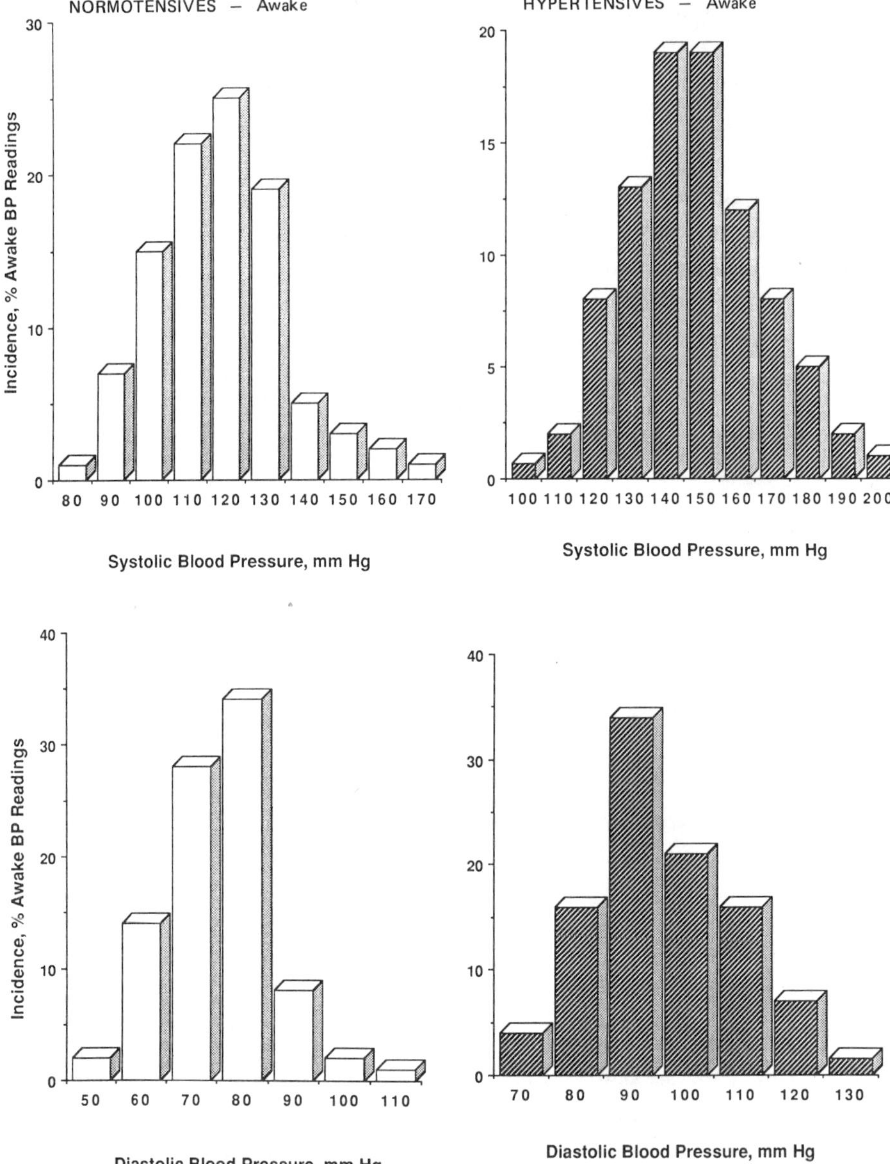

Figure 1.3 Distribution of awake blood pressures obtained by ambulatory monitoring in normotensives (open bars) and hypertensives (shaded bars). (Top) Systolic BPs; (bottom) diastolic BPs. (From White WB and Morganroth J, *Am J Cardiol* 1989, 63:94-98.

Table 1.2 Classification of Normotension and Hypertension in Adults (Based on Office or Clinic Measurements)

Blood (mm Hg) pressure range	Classification
DBP < 85	Normotension
DBP 85–89	High-normal BP
DBP 90–104	Mild hypertension
DBP 105–114	Moderate hypertension
DBP > 115	Severe hypertension
SBP < 140 and DBP < 90	Normotension
SBP 140–159 and DBP < 90	Borderline isolated systolic hypertension
SBP > 160 and DBP < 90	Isolated systolic hypertension

DBP, diastolic blood pressure; SBP, systolic blood pressure.
Source: Adapted from 1988 Joint National Committee Report, *Arch Intern Med* 1988;148:1023–1038.

by the 1988 Joint National Committee report (Table 1.2). While nearly all advice on the diagnosis and treatment of high blood pressure is based on diastolic pressure, there is substantial evidence from the Framingham study that systolic blood pressure is equal, if not superior, to diastolic blood pressure in predicting cardiovascular risk. There will be better guidelines on management of systolic hypertension when the results of SHEP (Systolic Hypertension in the Elderly Program) are available (see Chapter 3).

REFERENCES

Deubner D C, Tyroler H A, Cassel J C, Hames C G, Becker C. Attributable risk, population attributable risk, and population attributable fraction of death associated with hypertension in a biracial population. *Circulation* 1975;52:901-908.

Drayer J I M, Weber M A, Nakamura D K. Automated ambulatory blood pressure monitoring. A study in age-matched normotensive and hypertensive men. *Am Heart J* 1985;109:1334-1338.

1988 Joint National Committee. The 1988 report of the Joint National Committee on detection, evaluation, and treatment of high blood pressure. *Arch Intern Med* 1988;148:1023-1038.

Kannel W B, Sorlie P. Hypertension in Framingham. Second International Symposium Chicago Heart Association, in Paul O (ed): *Epidemiology and Control of Hypertension*. Symposia Specialists, New York; Stratton International Medical Book Co., Stuttgart, West Germany, 1975, pp. 553-555.

Mancia G, Grassi G, Pomidossi G, et al. Effects of blood pressure measurement by the doctor on patient's blood pressure and heart rate. *Lancet* 1983; 2:574-578.

Materson B J, Reda D, Freis E D, et al. Cigarette smoking interferes with treatment of hypertension. *Arch Intern Med* 1988; 148:2116-2119.

Medical Research Council Working Party. Stroke and coronary heart disease in mild hypertension: Risk factors and the value of treatment. *Br Med J* 1988; 296; 1565-1570.

Miall W E, Chinn S. Blood pressure and aging: results of a 15-17 year follow-up study in South Wales. *Clin Sci Mol Med* 1973; 45:235.

Murphy M B, Nelson K S, Oliner C M, Elliott W J. Higher nocturnal blood pressure in normal and hypertensive blacks compared with whites. *Circulation* 1988; 78:II-569.

Neaton J D, Kuller L H, Wentworth D, Borhani N O. Total and cardiovascular mortality in relation to cigarette smoking, serum cholesterol concentration, and diastolic blood pressure among black and white males followed up for five years. *Am Heart J* 1984; 108:759-769.

Pickering T G, James G D, Boddie C, Harshfield G A, Blank S, Laragh J H. How common is white coat hypertension? *JAMA* 1988; 259:225-228.

Svärdsudd K, Tibblin G. Mortality and morbidity during 13.5 years' follow-up in relation to blood pressure. *Acta Med Scand* 1979; 205:483-492.

White W B. Assessment of patients with office hypertension by 24-hour non-invasive ambulatory blood pressure monitoring. *Arch Intern Med* 1986; 146:2196-2199.

White W B, Morganroth J. Usefulness of ambulatory monitoring of blood pressure in assessing antihypertensive therapy. *Am J Cardiol* 1989; 63:94-98.

White W B, Schulman P, McCabe E J, Dey H M. Average daily blood pressure not office blood pressure determines left ventricular function in patients with hypertension. *JAMA* 1989, 261:873-877.

2

Evaluation of the Newly Diagnosed Hypertensive

I. MAKING THE DIAGNOSIS

Detection of an elevated blood pressure (BP) occurs in a variety of ways: during a routine annual physical examination or an emergency room or walk-in clinic visit for an unrelated problem, by an industrial nurse or doctor at the worksite, or from a BP screening conducted by a local health organization. However, the diagnosis of hypertension should not be made on the basis of a single BP measurement or even several measurements during one visit with the patient since this might lead to an inaccurate diagnosis.

There are a few situations that may uniformly lead to "higher than usual" BPs in susceptible individuals. For example, approximately half of the patients referred from emergency rooms to our hypertension unit for elevated BP readings have perfectly normal BPs recorded in visits at our office. Often the problem that brought them to the emergency room (ER) was some sort of minor trauma associated with considerable pain, and so even repeated BPs were elevated during their ER visit. Another typical example of episodic BP elevation is the young or middle-aged woman referred by a gynecologist following a routine examination and Papanicolau test because the nurse or doctor obtained a BP of, say, 150/95 mm Hg. The woman is referred to an internist—the less provoking examination with BP measurements, cardiopulmonary examination, and vascular evaluation does not incite the same anxiety as a gynecological examination and the result is a much lower BP of 115/75 mm Hg in the internist's office. Unfortunately, hypertension probably should not be diagnosed in the gynecologist's office even though he is usually the primary care physician for most young and many middle-aged women.

In any event, initially elevated BP readings should be confirmed on at least two subsequent visits, with average levels of systolic BP greater than 140 mm Hg and average levels of diastolic BP greater than 90 mm Hg. As mentioned in Chapter 1, these measurements should be performed in a seated position with the bare arm at heart level. It is important to ask the patient to refrain from smoking or drinking coffee or tea for the hour prior to the measurements.

In patients whose average BPs are in the moderate-to-severe range (diastolic BP > 105 mm Hg, systolic BP > 160 mm Hg), it is unlikely that manual home BP readings or even ambulatory BP measurements will yield additional information. However, it is still not unreasonable for interested patients to record BPs out of the office on a few occasions. In our experience, only about 5% of patients with moderately elevated office BPs (diastolic BPs, 105–114 mm Hg) have normal or borderline elevated BPs out of the doctor's office. On the other hand, in patients with borderline and mild hypertension (systolic BPs, 135–159 mm Hg, and diastolic BPs, 85–104 mm Hg), I strongly advise patients to purchase an inexpensive manual BP kit for out-of-office measurements. A nurse or assistant skilled in BP measurement should teach the patient the correct technique of BP measurement—we have employed a "teaching stethoscope," which allows the patient and nurse or doctor to listen to Korotkoff sounds simultaneously to make certain the patient understands how to correctly auscultate the first and last Korotkoff sounds.

Taking only home BPs while relaxed is not acceptable; patients must also record some BPs during work, if employed outside of the home. In about 80% of patients with mild hypertension, the out-of-office BPs will be within 5–10 mm Hg of the office BPs. We have not felt the need to perform ambulatory BP monitoring in patients whose office and out-of-office BPs are in close agreement with each other. Approximately 20% of patients whose BP is elevated in the doctor's office will have considerably different BPs from home and work (usually lower values outside the office). As mentioned in Chapter 1, it is now becoming increasingly common to perform automatic, noninvasive ambulatory BP monitoring in these individuals on a normal, working weekday. A practical problem in the past has been what to do with these new data—most clinicians do not have the background or the time to make an assessment of all the BPs from a 24-hr period. Fortunately, a number of investigators in the United States and Europe have been working on the "normalcy" of ambulatory BP, and while it is still not as solidly established in prognostic terms as office BP from the major epidemiological studies, it is quite useful for individual patients.

In Table 2.1, stepwise recommendations for confirming the diagnosis of hypertension are given once detection of an elevated BP reading occurs. These recommendations are the opinions of the author based on both the results from numerous studies and clinical experience. It has been recognized for some time by insurance actuarials that morbidity increases when the casual (office) diastolic BP is greater than 83 mm Hg. We don't call this hypertension, though, because we don't know how to effectively treat it. Since we are becoming increasingly aware of the lack of benefit of drug therapy in very mild hypertensives, a number of experts are not recommending initiating therapy (hence, confirming the diagnosis of hypertension) in patients who have diastolic BPs less than 95 mm Hg. The World Health Organization

Table 2.1   Recommended Steps for Diagnosing Hypertension

Average[a] office BP > 160/105 mm Hg: diagnosis of moderate or severe hypertension confirmed

Average office BP > 140/90 mm Hg and < 160/105 mm Hg: possible mild hypertension—obtain manual out-of-office BPs for several weeks

Manual home and work BPs average within 5–10 mm Hg of the office BPs: diagnosis of mild hypertension confirmed

Manual home and work BPs differ from office BPs by > 10 mm Hg: obtain ambulatory BP monitoring

Ambulatory BPs (awake) similar to office BPs, mean awake ambulatory BP > 135/85 mm Hg and 50% of awake readings > 140/90 mm Hg: patient is hypertensive

Ambulatory BPs (awake) < 135/85 mm Hg and 75% of awake readings are < 140/90 mm Hg and office BPs > 140/90 mm Hg: patient has "office" hypertension

25–50% of awake ambulatory BPs > 140/90 mm Hg: borderline hypertension

---

[a] Average is mean of three separate visits.

actually labels an individual hypertensive when the casual BP exceeds 160/95 mm Hg instead of the 140/90 mm Hg value recommended by the Joint National Committee on Detection, Evaluation, and Treatment of High Blood Pressure.

II. THE INITIAL WORKUP: SEARCHING FOR AN ETIOLOGY OF HYPERTENSION

In most published studies, only about 5% of all cases of hypertension have some specific cause even after thorough investigation. When no such cause can be found, hypertension is designated primary or essential, and then in patients who have a renal, endocrine, or drug-induced etiology, the term secondary hypertension is used. As will be discussed in subsequent chapters, the evaluation for secondary hypertension, especially renovascular disease, should be more aggressive in older hypertensive patients. On the other hand, the search for early signs of hypertensive heart disease should probably be more aggressive in younger hypertensive patients.

All patients with hypertension should have a complete history and physical examination. Historical questions of particular importance include details about past or present heart, renal, or vascular diseases, concomitant medical problems, and family history of high blood pressure, stroke, or coronary heart disease. Cardiac risk factor surveillance should be performed as well. It is useful to obtain information about cigarette, pipe, or cigar smoking; alcohol consumption; and prescription or recreational drug use. Failure to obtain these data could lead to an incorrect diagnosis that will last for a lifetime. As will be explained later, in Chapter 4, sometimes "resistance" is secondary to alcohol or drug abuse.

On physical examination, key areas of examination include the retina, peripheral blood vessels, heart and lungs, aorta, and extremities. Baseline findings such as arteriolar narrowing, diminished pulses or arterial bruits, a 4th heart sound, wheezing, a widened aorta, and peripheral edema have major impact on the diagnosis of hypertension as well as concerns about management. The presence of clear-cut target organ damage on physical examination undoubtedly changes the recommendations for diagnosis and initiating therapy made in Table 2.1. After all, if the patient already has signs of vascular disease from high blood pressure (assuming he or she does not have diabetes mellitus or hyperlipidemia), there is no reason to delay initiating therapy.

The extent of laboratory data required in the initial assessment of a hypertensive patient is a matter of controversy. If we assume that there has been no routine physical examination in the recent past, then the workup of the hypertension can be included in establishing a database. In general, the laboratory studies required to assess mild-to-moderate hypertension do not differ from those obtained in an annual complete physical examination (Table 2.2). Most clinicians agree on the need to obtain baseline hematological studies, urinalysis, electrolytes, blood glucose, renal function studies, uric acid, and a serum lipid profile. Tests that might be considered reasonable by some experts and quite extravagant by others include thyroid hormone studies, plasma or urinary

Table 2.2   Laboratory Studies Used in Baseline Assessment of Hypertension

---

Initial tests
   Complete blood count
   Urinalysis (dipstick and microscopic examination)
   Serum electrolytes, creatinine, uric acid, blood urea nitrogen
   Blood glucose
   Serum lipid profile (total and HDL cholesterol, triglycerides)
   12-lead electrocardiogram and rhythm strip
Special tests and indications
   Thyroid hormone levels (SBP high, DBP normal or low—suspect for hyperthyroidism)
   24-hr urine collection for catecholamines and/or metabolites (vanillylmandelic acid, normetanephrine)—suspect for pheochromocytoma
   Plasma renin activity/serum aldosterone (with serum/urine electrolytes)—hypokalemia—suspect for hyperaldosteronism
   M-mode and 2-D echocardiogram—younger hypertensives with borderline/ mild levels or patients with cardiac symptoms/signs
   Renal scan before and after captopril—suspect renovascular disease

---

HDL, high-density lipoprotein; SBP, systolic blood pressure; DBP, diastolic blood pressure.

catecholamines, plasma renin activity, and serum aldosterone. In our hypertension unit, we reserve all the latter tests for patients with severe hypertension, or for those in whom a particular clinical entity is suspected (e.g., symptoms of pheochromocytoma—catecholamines or unexplained hypokalemia—aldosterone).

In past years, obtaining a chest radiograph was strongly recommended by most organizations and experts dealing with hypertension as a routine part of the initial workup. However, there is little evidence that a chest X-ray is of benefit in the initial workup of hypertension, if the patient is a nonsmoker who has no pulmonary symptoms or abnormalities on physical examination. On electrocardiogram (ECG), a number of abnormalities can show up in patients with hypertension, including abnormal P waves from left atrial enlargement, left-axis deviation, increased voltage in the lateral precordial leads, and frank ST-T wave abnormalities associated with left ventricular hypertrophy (LVH). Less commonly seen are atrioventricular conduction disturbances. If there is interest in obtaining information about cardiac size though, the test of choice is an echocardiogram. While even a simple M-mode echocardiogram is twice as expensive as a posteroanterior and lateral chest film or an ECG, the information derived about the cardiac size and function is far superior to that obtained from either the chest film or ECG.

In many institutions in the United States, an echocardiogram is becoming a routine part of the diagnostic evaluation in younger and middle-aged patients with high blood pressure. The presence of LVH is an added risk factor for coronary heart disease and sudden death in patients with hypertension. Thus, in a patient with borderline elevations of the blood pressure who has mild LVH, early, rather than late, initiation of antihypertensive medication might be warranted.

The other special tests listed in Table 2.2 should probably be reserved for patients suspected to have a particular secondary form of hypertension. To simply order all of these studies in a patient with severe hypertension will not be practical or cost-effective, and 19 times out of 20, they will *all* be negative. In addition, some of the tests and their results are relatively complicated to obtain and interpret. For example, at most hospitals, the catecholamine studies—plasma epinephrine, norepinephrine, and dopamine—are sent to a central laboratory and you must wait several days to weeks for results. These studies are also quite expensive. Perhaps more important, the method of collection of plasma catecholamines is critical for the accuracy of the test. In most instances, the patient undergoing catecholamine studies should be untreated since many antihypertensive and cardiac drugs interfere with the assay or falsely elevate or lower the level of norepinephrine. Second, posture and the method of venipuncture are important since either can influence the levels of all three major catecholamine hormones. Central laboratories that perform these studies have standardized values for supine, seated, and standing levels of the hormones. It is generally a good idea to insert a heparin lock ('butterfly needle') about 30 min prior to obtaining the plasma sample and place the patient in the position that you wish to have the sample drawn at that time. This avoids a potential rise in norepinephrine or epinephrine secondary to pain or fear of pain from the needle stick—the fluctuations in these hormones are very rapid and pain, anxiety, or change in posture can induce an increase in catecholamines in a matter of minutes. Twenty-four-hour collections of urine for catecholamine metabolites (e.g., normetanephrine and vanillylmandelic acid) are more reproducible than episodic plasma sampling, but false elevations can still occur as a result of many of the antihypertensive drugs.

The methods of excluding renal artery stenosis and renovascular hypertension will be discussed more fully in Chapter 4. At the present time, radionuclide studies and angiography to rule out renal arterial disease are not considered part of the initial workup of mild-to-moderate hypertension in any age group other than infants and young children.

III. CONSIDERATIONS FOR STARTING THERAPY

Stratification by blood pressure level has been useful in the past, but we are realizing that the blood pressure alone does not provide adequate prognostic guidelines. Furthermore, in most instances, deciding on *what* class of drug to treat the patient with cannot be based just on blood pressure level or pathophysiology. Demographic characteristics and comorbid conditions are useful in decision making for initiating therapy. For example, blacks have more complications from hypertension, especially cerebrovascular disease and renal disease, than do whites. Men are at greater risk of coronary artery disease than women. Presumably a young patient with hypertension will be at risk for complications for a longer time than older patients with comparable blood pressure levels.

The presence of other known risk factors for coronary heart disease may also influence the decision to start therapy in patients with borderline or mild hypertension. Patients with mild hypertension who have elevations in low-density-lipoprotein cholesterol or reductions in high-density-lipoprotein cholesterol have a much greater likelihood of developing cardiovascular disease than individuals with normal lipid levels. As mentioned previously, individuals who smoke cigarettes dramatically increase their risk of heart and vascular diseases compared to nonsmokers with even considerably higher blood pressure. To a lesser degree, patients with other medical conditions such as diabetes mellitus, renal disease, or other types of heart disease are at a greater risk from their hypertension than those who are free of these conditions. Thus, these patients should be considered for earlier and more aggressive antihypertensive therapy (see Table 2.3).

Patients who have evidence on clinical or laboratory examination of end-organ involvement related to hypertension are at greater risk than individuals with similar blood pressure levels who are free of complications. In studies of mild-to-moderate hypertension where patients with prestudy target organ involvement were included (VA Cooperative Study and HDFP study), the benefit of therapy was much easier to demonstrate in those with prior target organ damage. But the risk of death from heart and vascular disease is almost four times as great if target organ damage is present at the time of diagnosis of hypertension. Thus, it is not ap-

Table 2.3 Characteristics of Borderline and Mild Hypertension that Favor Early Therapy

Demographic features—black patients, younger age, male sex
History of elevated LDL cholesterol or reduced HDL cholesterol
Cigarette smoking[a]
Evidence of target organ involvement—retinopathy, LVH on ECG or echocardiogram, proteinuria, diminished peripheral pulses
Strong family history of heart or vascular diseases
Coexisting medical illnesses—diabetes mellitus, other forms of heart or vascular diseases

[a]Cigarette smoking may interfere with the antihypertensive effects of the beta-adrenergic blocking agents.
LDL, low-density lipoprotein.
HDL, high-density lipoprotein.

propriate to consider any patient with elevated blood pressure and the presence of target organ involvement to have "mild" hypertension.

IV. INITIAL THERAPY OF HYPERTENSION

The entire gamut of nonpharmacological and pharmacological therapy cannot be reviewed here. At this point, salient features will be discussed regarding initial treatment in the mild-to-moderate, uncomplicated hypertensive patient. Subsequently, considerations for the management of special patient groups will be addressed at the end of each subsequent chapter.

A. Nonpharmacological Approaches

A number of modalities of nondrug therapies have been proposed, but few have proven efficacious, especially in long-term clinical studies (Table 2.4). Most nonpharmacological therapies of hypertension make practical sense though because they are associated with a healthy lifestyle. A moderate reduction in sodium intake to about 75–100 mEq (2–3 g) daily helps about one in four to five patients with hypertension but the reduction in BP is modest. Since there is no evidence that it is harmful to reduce sodium intake in the untreated patient, it is generally an acceptable first step

Table 2.4   Nonpharmacological Therapies in the Treatment of Hypertension

---

Efficacy documented in clinical trials
   Sodium restriction
   Reduction of body weight (if initially >25–30% above ideal)
   Restriction of alcohol to 2 oz daily
   Dynamic (or aerobic) exercise several times per week
Efficacy suggested in pilot studies (not proven in clinical trials)
   Supplementation of dietary potassium
   Supplementation of dietary calcium
   Supplementation of polyunsaturated fats
   Behavior modification, meditation, relaxation therapy

---

in managing borderline and mild hypertension with a nonpharma-cological method.

Weight loss can induce a dramatic BP reduction in many obese individuals with hypertension and should always be strongly advised. When patients are successful in losing weight and normal-izing their BP, they should still be closely followed. In our experi-ence, nearly every individual who regains the weight he lost will experience an increase in BP again—sometimes to even greater levels than observed previously.

Over the years, encouraging reports have shown reductions in BP following a regular dynamic exercise program. These are con-clusive studies which demonstrate that aerobic exercise, performed just three times per week (about 45–60 min each session) can re-duce resting BP in the absence of weight loss. Generally, there is a greater reduction in systolic pressure than diastolic pressure, as well as an expected fall in heart rate. Weight reduction and exer-cise have other obvious benefits for patients besides reducing BP, including lowering total cholesterol and raising high-density-lipo-protein cholesterol.

Unfortunately, the other nondrug approaches, both nutri-tional and behavioral, have not been proven efficacious conclusive-ly in long-term controlled studies (to my satisfaction). Thus, I can-not presently recommend them as a primary treatment of hyper-tension. Most physicians have seen patients who seem under un-usual duress and think that stress reduction may successfully re-duce the BP. Certainly a number of immediate and short-term studies suggest that relaxation therapy can modestly lower BP in some patients. However, the length of time that patients will comply with these types of behavioral therapy is highly variable, and to date no long-term studies (> 1 year) have reported on the effects of behavioral modification or relaxation therapy on a large cohort of hypertensives. For the present, the nutritional (exclud-ing restriction of sodium) and behavioral therapies can only be recommended as adjunct treatment to other nondrug or drug ther-apies of hypertension.

B. Drug Therapy

Rather than extensively discussing drug therapy in the present chapter, only general principles (Table 2.5) will be considered as specific agents are more useful than others in different types of patients. The studies of particular drugs or classes of drugs in different clinical situations, and their dosages, efficacy, and side effects, will be discussed in detail in chapters dealing with each specific type of hypertensive patient.

The best choices of initial antihypertensive therapy can be based on demographics, concomitant medical problems, cost, and previous or potential side effects. Another issue that may be important for our patients is the "protectiveness" or ability to prevent target organ involvement for a particular drug or class of drug. For example, in the patient with mild hypercholesterolemia and a family history of coronary heart disease, an agent that does not worsen the hyperlipidemia may be preferable to one that does increase cholesterol.

It is important to note that the most recent Joint National Committee Report (1988) does state that initial therapy could be with a variety of antihypertensive drugs, whereas in 1984, only diuretics and beta-adrenergic blocking drugs were used initially. In

Table 2.5   General Principles of Drug Therapy in the Initial Treatment of Essential, Uncomplicated Hypertension

---

Consider demographics, coexisting medical disorders, and cost of the medication

Take into account side effects from previous agents or potential side effects from a new drug

Appropriate first-line antihypertensive agents could include:
   angiotensin-converting enzyme (ACE) inhibitors
   beta-adrenergic blocking agents
   calcium channel blocking agents (long-acting)
   centrally acting alpha-2 agonists
   diuretics (preferably in patients with edema)
   peripheral alpha-1-adrenergic antagonists

---

recent years, in our hypertension unit, we have been using five classes of antihypertensives as monotherapeutic agents in mild, uncomplicated hypertension: (1) beta-adrenergic blocking agents (and alpha-beta blockers), (2) angiotensin-converting enzyme inhibitors, (3) long-acting calcium channel blockers, (4) centrally acting alpha-2 agonists, and (5) peripherally acting alpha-1-adrenergic blocking drugs. We have also used thiazide or loop diuretics as an initial therapy of mild hypertension but generally have preferred to use them in patients with edema. The diuretics certainly have been used for more than three decades as monotherapy for mild, essential hypertension, but at the present time, we have moved away from the use of the diuretics as monotherapy in uncomplicated hypertension. This decision has been based on accumulating data that show a lack of beneficial effects of the diuretics in reducing the risk of heart disease in hypertension, as well as their many numerous metabolic side effects, which require not only frequent laboratory monitoring, but dietary supplements of potassium and magnesium in more than 25% of the patients as well.

Finally, we address the pros and cons of the step-care approach to treating hypertension. Step-care therapy has been useful for the initial treatment of hypertension. It is easy to use, avoids the combination of inappropriate classes of drugs, and aids in the evaluation of drug resistance. However, there are certain drawbacks to the simple step-care therapy of hypertension. For example, it is possible that one might add a second drug to an initial therapy that had either very little or no effect on the level of the BP. Thus, the patient ends up taking two drugs instead of one. Excluding the technique of adding a second drug to an ineffective first drug and just substituting the second drug for the first drug is more appropriate in most cases. Another problem with step-care therapy is its lack of taking into consideration side effects from drugs which may seriously affect the quality of daily life. Since hypertension is basically an asymptomatic disease, using drugs that have few or no side effects has become preferable to using agents that make individuals feel far worse *on* therapy than they did when untreated.

REFERENCES

Ades, P A, Gunther P G S, Meacham C P, Handy M A, LeWinter M M. Hypertension, exercise and beta-adrenergic blockade. *Ann Intern Med* 1988; 109:629–634.

Black H R. Choosing initial therapy for hypertension—A personal view. *Hypertension*, 1989; 13 (suppl I):149–153.

Croog S H, Levine S, Testa M A, et al. The effects of antihypertensive therapy on the quality of life. *N Engl J Med* 1986; 314:1657–1664.

Kaplan N M. Non-drug treatment of hypertension. *Ann Intern Med* 1985; 102:359–373.

Joint National Committee Report on the Detection, Evaluation, and Treatment of High Blood Pressure. *Arch Intern Med* 1988; 148:1023–1038.

Lund-Johansen P. Treatment of essential hypertension today. *Med Clin North Am* 1987; 71:947–957.

3

The Elderly Hypertensive Patient

I. ILLUSTRATIVE CASE

A 74-year-old woman with a history of osteoarthritis had a blood pressure (BP) of 175/98 mm Hg on an annual physical examination. Her last recorded blood pressure was 155/88 mm Hg, 2 years earlier. A low-sodium diet was recommended at that time, and she had complied by avoiding salty processed foods as well as abstaining from using table salt. For nearly 6 years, she had been taking ibuprofen, 300 mg three times daily, with meals. She took no other prescription or over-the-counter medications, did not smoke, and drank a glass of wine about twice a week with dinner.

On physical examination, she was nonobese, had a heart rate of 68 bpm, average seated BP of 175/98 mm Hg, and standing BP of 165/102 mm Hg. Her funduscopic examination demonstrated arteriolar narrowing. Examination of the peripheral vessels disclosed a right femoral artery bruit. The cardiac examination revealed a 4th heart sound, and a harsh, grade II/VI midsystolic murmur heard best at the right sternal border, 2nd–3rd inter-coastal space. The remainder of the physical examination was normal.

Laboratory data showed a hemoglobin of 12.4 g/dl, hemato-crit of 36%, and normal white count and differential. The serum electrolytes were normal. The blood urea nitrogen was 14 mg/dl and serum creatinine, 0.7 mg/dl. Urinalysis showed a negative dip-stick examination; on microscopic examination of the urinary sed-iment, there were no cells, but a few hyaline casts were noted. Electrocardiogram showed a normal sinus rhythm at 65 beats/min. The P-R interval was 0.20 msec, the QRS interval was 0.11 msec, and there was a left-axis deviation of -45°. Because of the cardiac murmur and abnormal electrocardiogram, a Doppler echocardio-gram was ordered. This study demonstrated mild left concentric left ventricular hypertrophy with normal wall motion. The aortic valve had a moderate amount of calcification and the Doppler examination showed mild aortic insufficiency.

On a follow-up examination 2 weeks later, the average seated office BP was 178/100 mm Hg. Based on the BP level and findings on clinical examination suggesting target organ involvement from hypertension (retinal changes, femoral artery bruit, left ventricu-lar hypertrophy), a decision was made to begin drug therapy. The patient was unwilling to discontinue her ibuprofen as she had de-rived great benefit from this nonsteroidal antiinflammatory agent (NSAID) over the years. Thus, there were several issues to contend with in initial therapy in this particular patient, including her age, interaction with the ibuprofen, peripheral vascular disease, and borderline atrioventricular conduction times.

Her physician decided to initiate low doses of the angioten-sin-converting enzyme (ACE) inhibitor enalapril, 5 mg daily. Some of the considerations in the choice of initial therapy in this patient included the following: The drug works by lowering systemic vascular resistance, does not prolong atrioventricular conduction, and would not exacerbate the peripheral vascular disease. There have also been preliminary reports that the ACE inhibitors induce regression of left ventricular hypertrophy. Furthermore, there was concern that the hypotensive effects of the thiazide diuretics might have been attenuated by the NSAID (although the interaction may also occur with ACE inhibitors). The physician was also unwilling to begin a beta-adrenergic blocking drug as there were both prolonged P-R and QRS intervals. The other major classes of antihypertensives that could have been considered as initial therapy in this patient include the alpha-2 agonists (clonidine, guanabenz), the calcium channel blockers (nifedipine, nicardipine, diltiazem, verapamil), and the alpha-1 antagonists (prazosin, terazosin). The benefits and concerns about the various antihypertensive drugs in the elderly patient are discussed below.

II. CHARACTERISTICS OF THE ELDERLY HYPERTENSIVE

In most studies that characterize individuals as elderly, the minimum age for study entry has been either 60 or 65. Most of these same studies include either few or no patients over 70 or 80 years of age. Thus, the age ranges for most studies involving elderly hypertensives have been relatively narrow. In a discussion of the management of hypertension in the elderly, generalizations are often made that may not necessarily apply to individual patients. For example, the extent of the effects of aging on the heart and vascular tree may be far greater in a 65-year-old hypertensive individual who smoked cigarettes during his or her lifetime than in an 80-year-old nonsmoking hypertensive.

Age is probably one of our most important and reproducible clinical determinants of abnormal pathophysiology in a patient with hypertension. As shown by Lund-Johansen from Norway nearly 25 years ago, young patients with early essential hypertension are characterized by a normal vascular resistance while older patients have a high vascular resistance often accompanied by a depressed cardiac output (Fig. 3.1). These differences become even more marked during dynamic exercise, such as riding a bicycle. Thus, as time goes by the resistance in the blood vessels increases, and blood flow to important regional vascular beds, such as the heart, brain, kidneys, and intestines, falls. As the heart is working

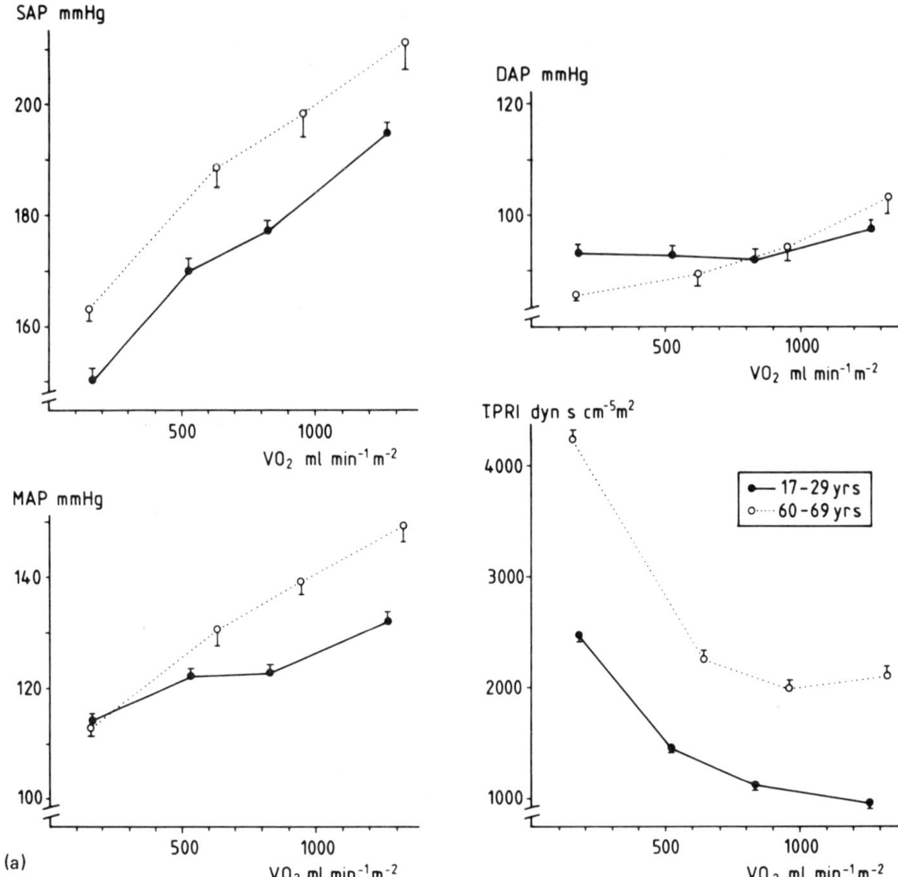

Figure 3.1 Contrasting hemodynamic patterns in early and late essential hypertension. SAP, systolic arterial pressure; DAP, diastolic arterial pressure; MAP, mean arterial pressure; HR, heart rate; TPRI, total peripheral resistance, indexed; CI, cardiac index; SI, stroke index. (From Lund-Johansen P, *J Cardiovasc Pharmacol* 1988; 12 (Suppl 8):S20–S30, with permission.)

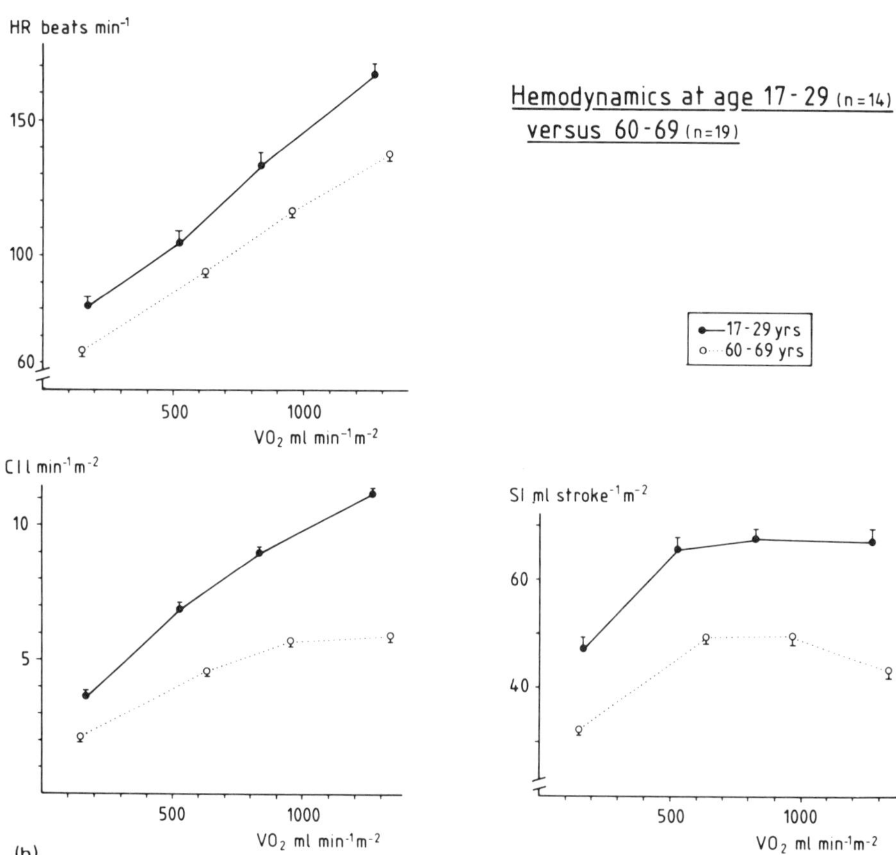

overtime against an increased resistance, the myocardium hypertrophies to overcome the chronic pressure overload. Unfortunately, left ventricular function worsens as this process continues for many years, since the myocardium becomes dysfunctional (especially during diastole) and fibrosis may develop.

Following the 5th decade, both systolic and diastolic blood pressures increase progressively with age; however, increases in systolic BP are more marked. An interesting example comes from a recent, longitudinal blood pressure study performed in Umbria,

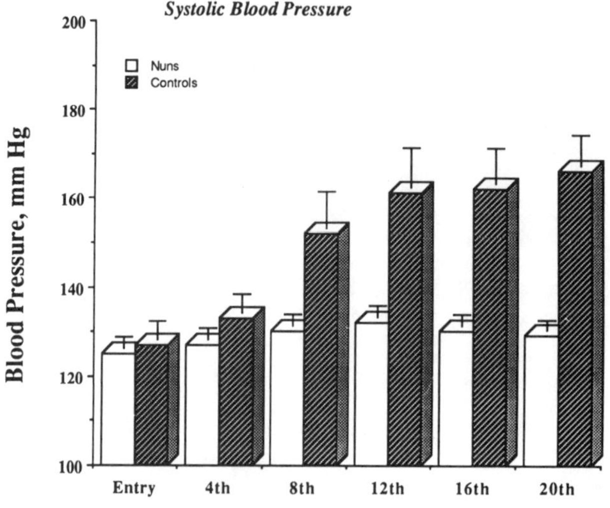

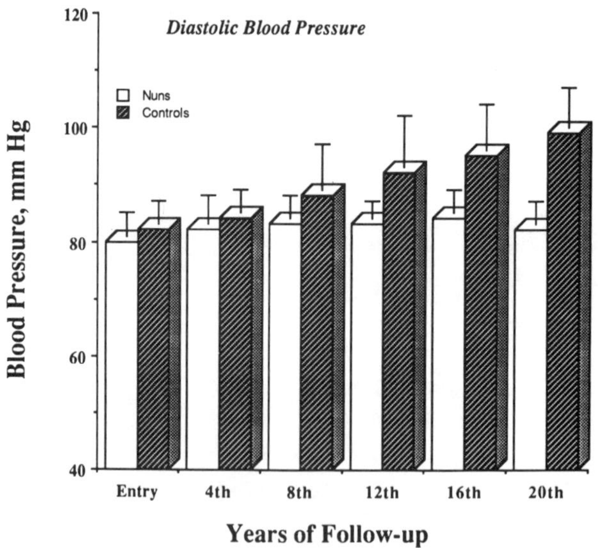

Figure 3.2   Systolic and diastolic blood pressure obtained every 4 years in nuns from a secluded order and age-matched controls. (From Timio M et al. *Hypertension* 1988; 12:457–461, with permission.)

Italy, with 144 nuns from a secluded order and a second group of age-matched women who were living typical suburban and rural lifestyles in Italy. The blood pressure increased impressively in the "control" group of women starting at about the age of 50, while almost no changes were seen in the nuns from the secluded order (Fig. 3.2). Other parameters, such as weight, cholesterol, renal function, and sodium excretion, were similar in both groups. Thus, one way of blunting the age-expected rise in blood pressure in women is to lead a monastic life.

In most surveys of blood pressure in the elderly, approximately 35–40% of Americans over 65 and under 75 have either an elevated systolic (>160 mm Hg) or diastolic (>90 mm Hg) BP, whereas another 8–10% have isolated systolic hypertension (ISH, defined as a systolic BP > 160 mm Hg and a diastolic BP < 90 mm Hg). If the threshold for diagnosis of isolated systolic hypertension was lowered to 140 mm Hg, then the incidence would likely triple to about 30% of the elderly population. Furthermore, the prevalence of ISH increases in individuals in their 80s and 90s. Unfortunately, these "age-related" changes in blood pressure cannot be considered a "normal" part of the aging process as they are associated with substantial increases in cardiovascular morbidity and mortality.

III. GUIDELINES FOR THE DIAGNOSIS OF HYPERTENSION IN THE ELDERLY

Different levels of systolic and diastolic blood pressure should probably not be used in elderly patients compared with younger patients when making the diagnosis of hypertension (Table 3.1). However, until more definitive data exist on benefits to the mildest subgroups of elderly hypertensives, it might be prudent to use modestly higher levels for initiating drug therapy. While there are a number of studies that suggest that BPs over 140/90 mm Hg are associated with an increase in stroke and myocardial infarction in older age groups, there are no available data from a controlled study that examined benefit of drug therapy in the milder forms

Table 3.1   Diagnosis of Hypertension in the Elderly

Borderline systolic hypertension—SBP > 140 but < 160 mm Hg with diastolic
   BPs < 90 mm Hg
Isolated systolic hypertension—SBP > 160 mm Hg and DBP < 90 mm Hg
Mild hypertension—both SBP > 160 mm Hg and DBP > 90 mm Hg but less
   than 180/105 mm Hg
Moderate hypertension—BP > 180/105 mm Hg but less than 200/115 mm Hg
Severe hypertension—BP > 200/115 mm Hg

SBP, systolic blood pressure; DBP, diastolic blood pressure.

of hypertension in the elderly. On the other hand, an intervention
trial known as the European Working Party on High Blood Pressure in the Elderly (EWPHE) has shown that in patients over 60
with moderate-to-severe hypertension (baseline BP in the group
was about 180/109 mm Hg), antihypertensive therapy was accompanied by impressive reductions in cardiovascular morbidity
and mortality. A philosophical debate has arisen as a result of that
trial; those *for treatment* (treatment of the elderly hypertensive
patient moderately reduced the risk of stroke), and those *against
treatment* (all-cause mortality was actually no different in the
treatment group versus the placebo group). Most clinicians agree
that treatment of moderate hypertension in the elderly is warranted if the risk of a cerebrovascular accident would be significantly reduced.

IV. SPECIAL FEATURES OF ELDERLY
PATIENTS WITH HYPERTENSION

Geriatricians have argued for years that older hypertensive patients
have a number of special physiological characteristics that must be
taken into consideration in their overall management (Table 3.2).
I agree with these specialists that we should keep these features
in mind when performing a physical examination on our older
hypertensive patients.

   Pseudohypertension is a fairly uncommon problem in older
hypertensive patients. The problem occurs when arteriosclerosis

Table 3.2   Special Physiological Features of Elderly Hypertensive Patients

Increased incidence of systolic (versus diastolic) hypertension
"Pseudohypertension" secondary to rigid peripheral arteries
Baroreceptor insensitivity (postural hypotension)
Abnormal cerebral blood flow autoregulation
Reduced glomerular filtration rate
"Stiff" left ventricle with diastolic dysfunction

causes the vessel wall to be too rigid for adequate occlusion by the sphygmomanometer cuff. The difference in the "externally" measured blood pressure from the direct or intraarterial blood pressure can be as great as 60/40 mm Hg. Pseudohypertension should be suspected in elderly patients who have stiff peripheral vessels and very high levels of blood pressure, but little evidence of vascular damage. Dr. Messerli and colleagues in New Orleans proposed a revival of the Osler maneuver in physical diagnosis: First one pumps up the sphygmomanometer cuff while palpating the radial artery on the same arm; if the radial pulse is still palpable after the Korotkoff sounds have disappeared over the brachial artery, then a large discrepancy (10–50 mm Hg) between the true intraarterial blood pressure and the cuff pressure is likely.

Another important physiological feature of older hypertensive patients is altered baroreceptor function. Elderly patients have reduced responsiveness of these pressure sensors, so that they are more susceptible to postural hypotension, postprandial falls in blood pressure, and occasionally, accentuated increases in blood pressure following various pressor stimuli. Taken together with reduced blood flow to the brain secondary to arteriosclerosis and/or disturbed cerebral blood flow regulation, elderly individuals may develop lightheadness or even syncope with postural blood reductions that would never have caused symptoms in a younger individual. Thus, enhanced orthostatic falls in blood pressure are commonly seen in elderly patients on many types of antihypertensive agents.

Glomerular function decreases progressively with age in normotensive subjects as well as hypertensive individuals. The commonly ordered renal function studies (urinalysis, serum electrolytes, creatinine, and blood urea nitrogen) often will miss reduced renal reserve. Remember that there can be a loss of as much as 50% of renal function before these tests are in an abnormal range. This is particularly important for considering drug therapy where an agent may be excreted by a renal mechanism or where an adverse effect of the drug includes some form of renal toxicity.

Over time, the function of the heart undergoes marked changes with hypertension and with aging. Sometimes it is not really possible to separate the effects of aging versus hypertension on cardiac function. Expected changes in the heart with aging include thickening of the ventricular walls, modest dilatation of the atria and ventricles, reduced diastolic filling rates, and impaired systolic responses to exercise. Pathological changes such as aortic stenosis and coronary artery disease may occur but may not be overtly symptomatic in elderly patients (these problems should be kept in the back of one's mind during the evaluation process).

V. SPECIAL PRACTICAL CONSIDERATIONS IN EVALUATION OF THE ELDERLY HYPERTENSIVE

In addition to the aforementioned physiological differences between older and younger hypertensive patients, there are also some practical clinical differences (Table 3.3). From the medical standpoint, there should be careful consideration of other disease processes, including peripheral vascular disease and congestive heart failure, diabetes mellitus, and arthritis. For example, if an elderly patient takes an NSAID for osteoarthritis, the clinician must bear in mind that there is a possible interaction of the NSAID with a variety of antihypertensive drugs. If the patient has clinically evident peripheral vascular disease, the goal BP of treatment should be modified to a higher level. If drug therapy reduces the systemic arterial pressure (measured in the arm) to 140/80 mm

Table 3.3 Practical Medical and Nonmedical Issues in the Assessment of Older Hypertensive Patients

---

Concomitant medical problems
  Peripheral vascular disease—goal of BP reduction should be modified to a higher level
  Diabetes mellitus—increased chance of renal disease, hyperkalemia, and intolerance of thiazide diuretics
  Arthritis—NSAIDs may interfere with antihypertensive drug effect
  Cerebrovascular disease—exaggerated postural hypotension
  Left ventricular hypertrophy ± CHF—impact on initial drug therapy
Practical nonmedical issues
  Multiple medications (nonantihypertensives and antihypertensives)—confusion in what does what; potential side effects
  Limited income and insurance coverage—cost containment may be critical in these situations
  Difficulty with travel to have blood pressure checks or doctor's visits

---

CHF, congestive heart failure.

Hg, it may also be reducing the blood pressure in the foot from 90/60 mm Hg to 50/30 mm Hg and rest pain will develop. Most clinicians are aware that diabetic hypertensives are more likely to have renal insufficiency but in addition, they are more likely to have mild hyperkalemia since older diabetic patients develop hyporeninemic hypoaldosteronism and have reduced excretion of potassium.

A number of elderly patients with hypertension have had a transient ischemic attack or a stroke. These patients are more likely to have had a thrombotic stroke than a hemorrhagic stroke, as mentioned in Chapter 1. Thus, there must be some caution in initiating therapy and in deciding the type of therapy in these individuals as well. Furthermore, the long-term association of hypertension and cerebrovascular accidents should be discussed with the patient since it is commonly thought (by patients) that even moderate levels of blood pressure elevation can cause an acute stroke.

Many of my elderly patients take a great deal of medication for conditions other than hypertension or cardiovascular disease. Some of these medications are as expensive as their antihypertensive drugs and some are quite a bit less. Nevertheless, many elderly patients have a difficult time affording their monthly medication bill, especially when insurance coverage is minimal and income is limited. Therefore, the cost of the medication should be addressed with all patients—I find it useful to find out what a patient's monthly medication bill is. It is not uncommon to find some patients spending $200 per month for medications while they are receiving $800 per month through social security payments. Furthermore, it is useful to recommend that patients survey several local pharmacies for large differences in prices—we have noted 20–30% differences in trade-name antihypertensive drugs in pharmacies not more than 3 miles apart from each other!

VI. INITIAL THERAPY OF THE ELDERLY HYPERTENSIVE

A. Nonpharmacological Therapy

It is reasonable to consider nonpharmacological treatment of elderly hypertensives, especially if the elevation of blood pressure is mild or only the systolic pressure is elevated. Dietary measures (especially reduction of salt and calories) are the most commonly advocated nondrug treatment of the elderly. They may work in a small percentage of patients, but our experience has been that dietary restriction of salt is less effective in elderly patients than in younger individuals even though compliance may be fairly good. Restricting calories in obese older patients may also be beneficial in reducing the blood pressure but care should be taken in advising the elderly to ensure that the new diet is nutritionally adequate.

B. General Considerations for Drug Therapy

If nondrug therapy is not successful, then drug therapy should be initiated. As mentioned above (Table 3.2), there are a number of special physiological features of the elderly hypertensive which must be kept in mind before starting antihypertensive agents. The reduced plasma volume, decreased baroreceptor sensitivity, and propensity for postural hypotension may make older individuals more susceptible to the blood-pressure-lowering effects of these drugs. I think it reasonable to start all antihypertensive drugs in the elderly at *half* the dose I would use in a younger patient. In addition, it is a good idea to advance the dose more gradually, checking carefully for the presence of postural hypotension at all visits.

C. The Diuretics

Some hypertension experts consider the diuretics to be the best agents for initial therapy in elderly hypertensive patients. There are quite a bit of data demonstrating the efficacy of the thiazide diuretics in geriatric hypertension trials. Using a dose equivalent to 12.5–25 mg of hydrochlorothiazide lowered BP by about 30/15 mm Hg in the EWPHE study although those patients did start out at a fairly high pretreatment blood pressure (the higher the pretreatment blood pressure, the greater the blood pressure fall with therapy). However, in the pilot study of the Systolic Hypertension in the Elderly Program (SHEP), a low-dose diuretic controlled about 85% of the patient's systolic BP (< 160 mm Hg) for the year of the study.

The most controversial issue about diuretics is their safety in the elderly (Table 3.4). Perhaps the most serious side effect is

Table 3.4   Adverse Effects of the Diuretics and Symptoms Associated with Them

Hyponatremia—confusion, lethargy, convulsions
Prerenal azotemia—postural hypotension, lethargy
Hypokalemia—muscle weakness/cramps, arrhythmias (rare)
Glucose intolerance—symptoms associated with diabetes
Hyperuricemia—gout, renal calculi
Hyperkalemia/hyponatremia—when potassium-sparing agents are used in conjunction with a thiazide or loop diuretic

hyponatremia, which occurs in about one of six elderly individuals taking diuretics. While severe cases of hyponatremia are rare, they are associated with confusion, convulsions, Stokes-Adams attacks, and even death. In elderly patients whom it is deemed necessary to maintain on a diuretic despite mild hyponatremia, liberalization of salt intake helps in normalizing the serum sodium. Another important side effect of diuretics in the elderly is prerenal azotemia, which occurs, in part, secondary to a diminished renal reserve in the older individuals.

The diets of elderly patients are more likely to lack fruits and vegetables, especially if these patients are widowed. Therefore, these patients are particularly susceptible to potassium deficiency associated with an oral diuretic. The incidence of hypokalemia in the elderly taking diuretics is around 5–10%. The problem of muscle cramps and weakness is seen when the potassium level is very marginally depressed, but it is quite subjective, and studies of the relationship between muscle weakness and serum potassium are inconclusive. The most serious consequence of hypokalemia is cardiac arrhythmia, but this is relatively rare unless the potassium level has fallen below 3.0 mEq/liter or the patient is concomitantly taking a digitalis preparation. While potassium-sparing agents (e.g., triameterene, spironlactone, and amiloride) are more expensive than generic diuretics, many clinicians tend to use them in combination with the thiazide rather than potassium supplements. Since one needs to give substantial amounts of potassium (20–30 mEq daily) to replace what is lost by the effects of the thiazide, the price differential may not be that great. When a potassium-sparing agent is used, monitoring of the serum potassium is just as important as ever, since some elderly patients (especially those with reduced renal function) could develop hyperkalemia.

A more overt side effect of the diuretics in elderly women and men is precipitation of the gout, especially podagra. The serum level of uric acid may not even be in the hyperuricemic range when these symptoms develop. Finally, a relatively well-known metabolic consequence of the diuretics is worsened glucose tolerance. Sometimes we see elderly patients developing overt

symptoms of diabetes mellitus associated with pronounced increases in the blood glucose following initial therapy with a thiazide diuretic. For the most part, though, there is an asymptomatic
rise in blood sugar, with occasional development of glycosuria.

The loop diuretics (bumetanide, ethacrynic acid, and furosemide) are not appropriate as first-line antihypertensive agents in
the elderly, with two exceptions: first, if the renal reserve is
markedly diminished to a creatinine clearance of under 20 ml/min,
and second, if there is concomitant congestive heart failure that is
refractory to a thiazide diuretic. The efficacy of the loop diuretics
is not any greater than that of a thiazide diuretic in uncomplicated
hypertension unless these concomitant problems exist. On the
other hand, most of the side effects, such as volume depletion,
hyponatremia, and hypokalemia, are greater with the loop
diuretics.

D. Beta-adrenergic Blocking Agents

In 1984, the Joint National Committee added the nine available
beta-blocking agents to diuretics as first-line therapy in the treatment of hypertension. In 1988, the angiotensin-converting enzyme
inhibitors and calcium channel blockers were added to the classes
of antihypertensive agents that were appropriate first-line drugs.
However, as recently as 1986, the Working Group on Hypertension in the Elderly commented that the beta-blockers were not
first-line drugs in treating hypertension in the elderly because
these patients were relatively resistant to monotherapy with these
agents. Apparently, this recommendation was based more on theoretical grounds than on clinical research findings. A large international study was performed from the mid-1970s until the mid-
1980s comparing hydrochlorothiazide versus the beta-blocking
drug metoprolol in patients aged 60–75 years, as reported in 1986
by Wikstrand and co-workers. The major finding was that metoprolol was equal in efficacy to the diuretic and had a similar incidence of adverse side effects. As would be expected, more patients
in the diuretic group had reduced serum potassium and increased
serum uric acid compared to the beta-blocker monotherapy group.

The beta-blocking drugs are particularly useful antihypertensive agents in elderly patients who have coronary heart disease, including those with angina pectoris or a previous myocardial infarction. They can be used alone or in combination with a diuretic, if blood pressure control is not satisfactory with the beta-blocking drug alone. Side effects to be expected with the use of beta-blockers in the elderly are not really different from those in a younger population. Actually, the beta-blockers induce less postural hypotension than many other classes of antihypertensive agents and, thus, may have potential benefit in elderly individuals prone to postural hypotension. In the study noted above, the most common side effects from metoprolol included headaches, sleep disturbances, the gastrointestinal symptoms. If more lipid-soluble drugs are used, such as propranolol or timolol, nightmares and depression may be more common. One important finding in studies of beta-blockers in uncomplicated, elderly hypertensive patients is a remarkably low incidence of development of congestive heart failure. As a word of caution, though, patients should be carefully evaluated before starting treatment with beta-blockers to exclude possible contraindications such as left ventricular systolic dysfunction, bradycardia, heart block, or bronchospasm.

E. Angiotensin-Converting Enzyme Inhibitors

The safety and efficacy of the ACE inhibitors, (captopril, enalapril, and lisinopril) have been reported only in short-term studies in elderly patients. There is really no reason to expect development of tolerance (hence, reducing efficacy) or that a serious ACE inhibitor adverse side effect will develop if these problems did not occur in the first several weeks of treatment, however. In a fairly well-done study with captopril in a patient population averaging 66 years, efficacy was satisfactory over an 8-week period of observation and side effects were relatively few in number.

The ACE inhibitors may be particularly beneficial for elderly hypertensive patients who also have congestive heart failure. Indeed, they may be the drugs of choice in these individuals. The hemodynamic properties of the ACE inhibitors include a reduc-

Table 3.5 Antihypertensive Drug Therapy for Hypertension in the Elderly

Agent	Special benefits	Common side effects
ACE inhibitors	Hemodynamic effect is appropriate; useful in CHF patients	Cough, rash, taste dysfunction, worsened GFR in patients with renal disease
Beta-blockers	Effects on coronary disease	Fatigue, bradycardia, bronchospasm
Calcium channel blockers	Hemodynamic profile, effects on coronary disease	AV block (V), constipation (V), flushing edema (N)
Centrally acting alpha-agonists	Proven efficacy, no effect on cerebral blood flow	Multiple CNS side effects
Peripheral alpha-antagonists	Effective in isolated systolic hypertension	Postural hypotension
Thiazide diuretics	Proven efficacy	Multiple metabolic side effects

AV, atrioventricular; CHF, congestive heart failure; CNS, central nervous system; GFR, glomerular filtration rate; N, nifedipine; V, verapamil.

tion in both afterload (systemic vascular resistance) and preload (venodilation with reduced atrial pressure). A *word of warning*: a fairly high percentage of older hypertensive patients (10–20%) have significant aortic and renal arterial atherosclerosis. If these individuals have bilateral renal disease with reduced intrarenal blood flow, an ACE inhibitor may markedly reduce the glomerular filtration rate and even cause oliguria. Careful clinical examination prior to initiating drug therapy, including evaluation for peripheral vascular disease, auscultating for renal artery bruits, palpating the aorta, and assessing renal function, will aid in avoiding inappropriate use of an ACE inhibitor in an elderly patient.

F. Calcium Channel Blocking Agents

For many years prior to their approval for the treatment of hypertension in the United States, the calcium channel blockers were touted abroad as superior initial agents for the elderly population. As the elderly have an increased systemic vascular resistance

(SVR) often accompanied by a low cardiac output (Fig. 3.1), the calcium channel blockers can be quite efficacious in lowering blood pressure by markedly reducing SVR while having no effect on cardiac output. In young patients with hypertension, a known side effect of vasodilators, including the calcium channel blockers, is reflex sympathetic stimulation of the heart. Fortunately, older patients rarely experience this problem because of a blunted autonomic nervous system associated with reduced adrenergic receptor sites. Thus, the calcium channel blockers, diltiazem, nifedipine, nicardipine, and verapamil-SR, can all be potentially used as monotherapies in the treatment of hypertension in the elderly.

There are some disadvantages to the calcium channel blockers in older hypertensive patients; however, they are relatively minor. At the present time (1989), only verapamil-SR is a once-daily agent, while the others must be given two or three times per day to achieve adequate blood pressure control. Long-acting preparations of diltiazem and nifedipine are soon to be available, however. Verapamil-SR is notorious for inducing constipation in about 20–25% of older hypertensive patients but it is related to the dose level and generally worse in patients who are prone toward constipation in the first place. On a more serious note, uncomplicated elderly hypertensives rarely develop atrioventricular conduction disturbances (e.g., junctional rhythm, complete heart block) on larger doses of verapamil. In patients taking a digitalis preparation, one has to be careful with both verapamil and diltiazem, since the combination of either of these calcium channel blockers with digoxin can induce bradycardia.

G. Centrally Acting Alpha Agonists

The alpha-2 agonists, clonidine, guanabenz, and methyldopa, also work well in the elderly since they lower blood pressure by reducing SVR. The efficacy of the centrally acting alpha agonists has been established for a long time in the elderly population since these drugs have been available for many years in the United States. There is a theoretical benefit to the use of these drugs in the elderly since they do not reduce regional blood flow, notably in the cerebral and renal vascular beds. On the other hand, side effects are relatively common with the alpha-2 agonists and include drowsiness, dry mouth, and occasionally confusion. A transdermal preparation of clonidine (TTS-clonidine) can be used once a week and may improve compliance and lessen the side effects compared to the oral forms of the alpha-2 agonists.

H. Peripheral Alpha-1 Antagonists

The peripheral alpha-blockers include prazosin, terazosin, and labetalol (which actually has multireceptor blocking properties as an alpha-beta blocker). These drugs are effective at lowering systolic blood pressure in patients with isolated systolic hypertension. Sometimes they are effective when no other drug works. However, the incidence of postural hypotension associated with the alpha-1 antagonists is substantial in the elderly and not uncommonly causes syncope. Because of this rather serious side effect, I do not consider the alpha-1 antagonists a first-line monotherapy in elderly hypertensive patients. If they must be used because of refractory systolic hypertension, minimal initial doses should always be given.

I. Combination Therapy

Many of the previously listed drugs can be used in combination if control of the blood pressure is not established with a single agent from one of the six classes listed above. An additive effect can be expected when diuretics are added to the beta-blockers, calcium channel blockers, ACE inhibitors, centrally acting alpha-2 agonists, and peripheral alpha-1 antagonists. However, postural hypotension may be exaggerated with vasodilators in patients who are moderately volume-depleted from the diuretics. Beta-adrenergic blocking agents can be combined safely with ACE inhibitors or calcium channel blocking agents as well, but this is a costly combination. It is not generally a good idea to combine two different sympatholytic drugs in an elderly patient since the potential for lethargy, confusion, and depression would be moderately increased. The combination of ACE inhibitors and calcium channel blockers is relatively powerful in the elderly and again relatively expensive. Finally, using an ACE inhibitor with an alpha-blocker is also a potent combination but again fairly likely to exaggerate the possibility of postural hypotension—thus, I would reserve this combination for the most severe cases and use it with great caution in an elderly individual.

REFERENCES

Amery A, Brixko P, Clement D, et al. Mortality and morbidity results from the European Working Party on High Blood Pressure in the Elderly Trial. *Lancet* 1985; 1:1349-1354.

Hla K M, Feussner J R. Screening for pseudohypertension. *Arch Intern Med* 1988; 148:673-676.

Lund-Johansen P. The hemodynamics of the aging cardiovascular system. *J Cardiovasc Pharmacol* 1988; 12 (Suppl 8):S20-S30.

MacLennan W J. Diuretics in the elderly: how safe? *Br Med J* 1988; 296: 6636.

Messerli F H, Ventura H O, Amodeo C. Oster's maneuver and Pseudohypertension. *N Engl J Med* 1985; 312:1548-1551.

Radin A M, Black H R. Hypertension in the elderly: The time has come to treat. *J Am Geriatr Soc* 1981; 29:193-200.

Timio M, Verdecchia P, Venanzi S, et al. Age and blood pressure changes: A 20-year follow-up study in nuns in a secluded order. *Hypertension* 1988; 12:457-461.

Tuck M L, Katz L A, Kirkendall W M, et al. Low-dose captopril in mild to moderate geriatric hypertension. *J Am Geriatr Soc* 1986; 34:693-696.

Wikstrand J, Westergren G, Berglund G, et al. Antihypertensive treatment with metoprolol or hydrochlorothiazide in patients aged 60 to 75 years. *JAMA* 1986; 255:1304-1310.

Working Group on Hypertension in the Elderly. Statement on Hypertension in the Elderly. *JAMA* 1986; 256:70-74.

4

Evaluation and Treatment of the Resistant Hypertensive

I.   WHO IS A RESISTANT HYPERTENSIVE?

The term "resistant" or "refractory" hypertensive has been used for many years to describe "problem" patients whose blood pressure (BP) is either unusually difficult to bring under control or perhaps even impossible to normalize with the available therapy. Classically, resistant hypertension was used to describe patients who had failed to achieve a normal office or clinic BP ($<140/90$ mm Hg) despite standard triple-drug therapy with a diuretic, sympatholytic agent, and direct vasodilator. The advent of new classes of antihypertensive drug therapy over the last decade, such as angiotensin-converting enzyme inhibitors and the calcium channel blockers, has made drug-resistant hypertension much less common than it was prior to the mid-1980s. Nevertheless, these patients are problematic, and I am well aware that most internists and family practitioners encounter difficult-to-control patients regularly since the resistant hypertensives have actually formed a consultative practice for me.

In practical terms, there is no precise blood pressure level before and during treatment that defines a patient with resistant hypertension. In the literature, however, most hypertension experts suggest that resistant (or refractory) hypertension be defined when patients with severe hypertension (BP > 180/115 mm Hg prior to treatment) fail to achieve stable, controlled BP with maximal doses of two- or three-drug regimens. I have chosen to continue to use these criteria as a working definition for resistant hypertension. However, it is reasonable to allow some flexibility in the diagnosis since, as subsequently noted in this chapter, the causes of drug-resistant hypertension are varied.

II. ILLUSTRATIVE CASES

A. Renovascular Hypertension

A 48-year-old woman presented to her general internist because of asymptomatic, but severe hypertension. At a recent BP screening program, her BP level was 200/115 mm Hg. This was a great surprise to her since just 2 years earlier an annual physical examination yielded an office BP of 115/80 mm Hg. On physical examination, her office BP averaged 200/110 mm Hg and the heart rate was 72 beats/min. Funduscopic examination revealed no retinopathy. On cardiac examination, a 4th heart sound was auscultated but all else was normal. Initial laboratory data, including urinalysis, serum electrolytes, uric acid, creatinine, glucose, and blood urea nitrogen, were normal. An electrocardiogram showed no evidence of left ventricular hypertrophy, conduction abnormalities, or ischemia. Her physician chose hydrochlorothiazide (25 mg daily) as the initial medication along with a low-salt diet. Following 1 month of therapy, the BP was 180/105 mm Hg. This was considered a partial response, so a second drug, atenolol (50 mg daily), was added. Over the next several weeks, even with an increase of the atenolol to 100 mg daily and reduction in resting heart rate to 60 beats/min, the BP did not change.

By this time, the patient felt certain that her BP was elevated secondary to a busy, stressful lifestyle. Her home BPs (taken manually by herself) were almost identical to the measurements obtained in the doctor's office. She rarely, if ever, drank alcohol, and did not smoke cigarettes. She was appropriately concerned about her hypertension and appeared to be compliant in taking the hydrochlorothiazide and atenolol regularly. After consultation, in the hypertension unit, we initiated enalapril, 5 mg daily, as a third agent. In 1 week, the office and home BPs were in the range of 130–140/80–90 mm Hg.

A renal digital subtraction arteriogram was performed and showed a nearly occluded midsection of the right renal artery (Fig. 4.1) secondary to fibromuscular hyperplasia. The left renal artery, aorta, and iliac arteries were normal and free of atherosclerotic plaque. Since she had a triad of severe hypertension, a marked unilateral renal artery stenosis, and a positive hemodynamic response to an ACE inhibitor, percutaneous transluminal angioplasty (PTCA) was performed at the same time as the arteriogram. The vessel was opened to its normal size and blood flow was restored to the right kidney (Fig. 4.2).

Within a few hours of the procedure, the BP fell to 105/60 mm Hg and all antihypertensives were withheld in the hospital. Three days later, she was discharged with a BP of 115/70 mm Hg. Antihypertensive medications were never restarted, and nearly 2 years after the PTCA, this patient remains normotensive.

B. Office Hypertension

A 28-year-old man presented to our clinic when his family doctor became concerned that his BP control remained inadequate despite multiple types of medication over the previous 6 months. He had presented for a preemployment examination and was found to be hypertensive (BP, 160/102 mm Hg). There were no symptoms of any sort. On two subsequent visits, the hypertension was confirmed, routine physical examination and laboratory tests were negative, and the physician started the patient on long-acting propranolol, 60 mg daily. Within a few days, the patient complained of fatigue and low energy levels. The long-acting pro-

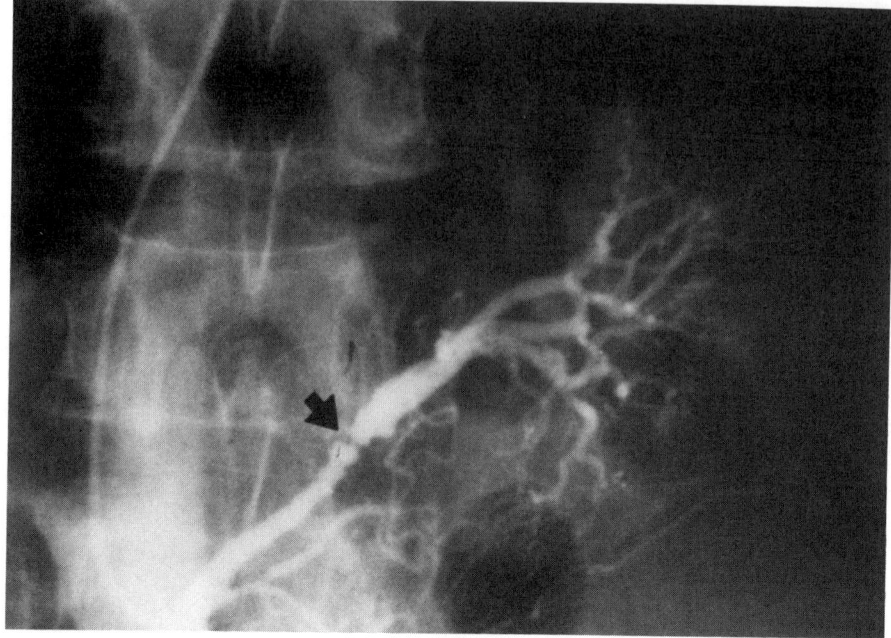

Figure 4.1 Selective right renal arteriogram showing a tight midvessel stenosis with the 'beading' characteristic of fibromuscular hyperplasia.

pranolol was promptly discontinued, and enalapril, 5 mg daily, was initiated. The company nurse measured the patient's BP twice a week for the next month and obtained levels in the vicinity of 145/100 mm Hg. In the family practitioner's office, the BP was usually 155–165/100–105 mm Hg even with doses of enalapril of

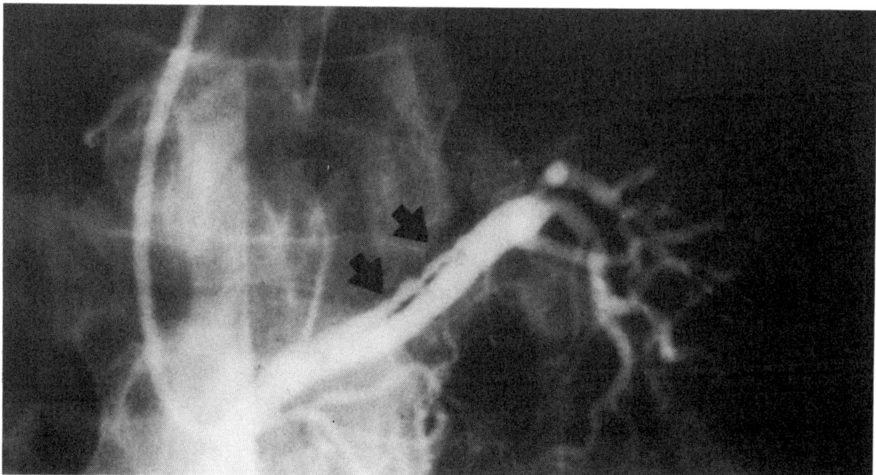

Figure 4.2   Renal arteriogram following angioplasty shows restoration of flow and normal lumen size.

up to 20 mg daily. The doctor added a small dose of a thiazide diuretic, 12.5 mg daily, to the enalapril.

Two weeks later the patient began to experience occasional lightheadedness at noon but often felt a little better after he ate lunch. The nurse at his factory measured BPs of approximately 135–140/90–95 mm Hg; in the physician's office, the readings were about 5 mm Hg higher. Soon thereafter, the patient had a 24-hr urine collection for catecholamine metabolites and a renal isotope scan. Both of these studies were normal. The enalapril was

Table 4.1   Flow Sheet of Manual Blood Pressures for Patient 2

Date	Place	Time	Blood pressure	Pulse rate
5/3	Home	6 p.m.	125/78 mm Hg	Not done
5/4	Home	4 p.m.	112/78 mm Hg	68 bpm
5/5	Work	11 a.m.	130/85 mm Hg	74 bpm
5/6	Work	12 p.m.	135/86 mm Hg	74 bpm
5/7	Home	8 p.m.	128/90 mm Hg	72 bpm
5/8	Home	7 a.m.	120/68 mm Hg	64 bpm
5/9	Work	10 a.m. (nurse)	140/88 mm Hg	76 bpm

discontinued and verapamil in sustained-release tablets was started at 240 mg daily. Over the next 4–6 weeks, the BP still remained in the 140/90–95 mm Hg range.

Some of our first questions to this young man included inquiries about alcohol consumption, compliance with his medications, and whether he monitored his own BP. He stated he drank only one glass of wine at dinner, that he never missed his BP pills, and that he did not take his BP as the nurse at work usually did that. The BP we obtained in the clinic was approximately 165/105 mm Hg. Clinical evaluation did not show any signs of overt target organ damage. We suggested that he purchase an inexpensive aneroid manometer, come for a training session with our nurse, and begin to monitor his own BP. Table 4.1 is a flow sheet for his home and work BPs for the first week.

After reviewing the flow sheet, we decided to perform 24-hr ambulatory BP monitoring on his usual drug regimen of hydrochlorothiazide and verapamil, sustained-release tablets. As shown in Figure 4.3, the BP was almost always under 140/90 mm Hg while awake and dropped to levels of only about 100/60 mm Hg while he slept. A few readings were taken in the hospital going to and from the hypertension unit and in the presence of the doctor

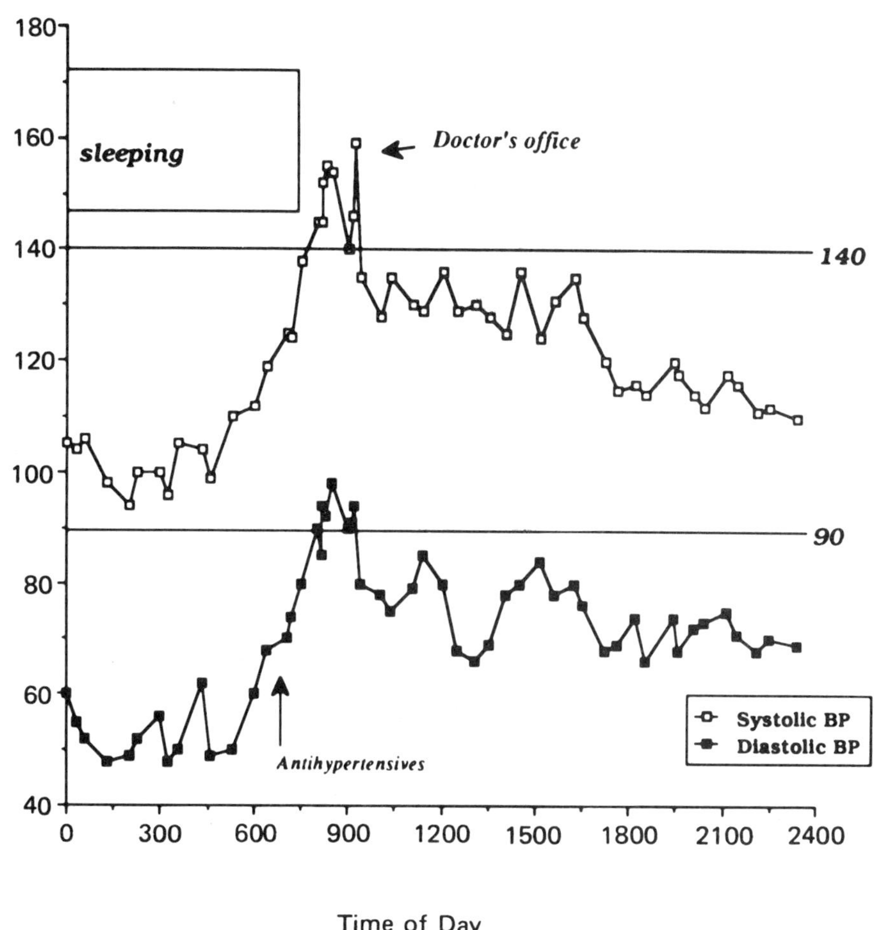

Figure 4.3 Twenty-four-hour blood pressure profile in patient 2—a young man who had hypertension only in the medical care environment.

and these constituted the only truly hypertensive readings of the day. So despite antihypertensive medications, this patient developed enough of a pressor response in the presence of a doctor or nurse to appear to be poorly controlled. On the earlier regimen that included enalapril, 20 mg daily, it is likely that the patient was experiencing overshoot hypotension in the middle of day when the drug has its peak effect. While not shown in Figure 4.3 (since his drug had been changed by then), ambulatory blood pressure monitoring could have been useful in detecting this type of phenomenon.

A few weeks later the patient was evaluated with 24-hr ambulatory BP monitoring on verapamil monotherapy and found to have normotensive out-of-office BP values. After nearly 1 year of seeing his physician regularly, he has lower (but not yet normal) blood pressures.

III. CAUSES OF RESISTANT HYPERTENSION

A. Compliance

The cases above were two quite different, but common examples of resistant hypertension. When one encounters a patient whose blood pressure is difficult to control, it is reasonable to consider a secondary form of hypertension or some other underlying etiology (e.g., office hypertension) (Table 4.2). At the outset, it is

Table 4.2   Causes of Resistant Hypertension

Patient noncompliance
Various types of secondary hypertension
  Renovascular hypertension (renal artery stenosis)
  Hyperaldosteronism (adrenal adenoma or hyperplasia)
  Pheochromocytoma (rare)
Office or white-coat hypertension
Alcohol excess
Drug abuse (cocaine, amphetamines)
Drug interactions/antagonism

important to verify that the patient is compliant with his medications. Fortunately, it is uncommon that patients attempt to deceive a physician into thinking they are taking medications when they are not. However, it is not unusual that several doses of a drug (especially those that are administered twice or thrice daily) are missed during the course of a week. Several years ago, I participated in a study in which a new beta-adrenoreceptor blocking agent assay was being validated. We obtained plasma concentrations on 50 patients who had been taking the beta-blocker atenolol for a minimum of 3 months. To my surprise, about 15% of the patients had levels of <5 ng/ml (or next to nothing!). When we called these patients to ask about their compliance, since the concentration of the drug in their plasma was close to zero, they all admitted to frequently "forgetting" to take their pills.

It is neither practical nor possible to obtain drug concentration levels on patients in clinical practice. Other, more practical maneuvers have been used to aid in assessing compliance in our clinic. For example, we ask patients to recall the names of all their medications, the dose, and what they look like (many doctors don't know what the medications look like but you'll soon learn—the *Physicians' Desk Reference* is quite helpful in this regard). On the day of their appointment, we always ask patients what *time* they took their antihypertensive medications that day (this also helps in assessing whether we are seeing a peak or trough dose response). Finally, we have a clinical pharmacist who interviews our patients briefly and directly discusses compliance issues. In private practice, a nurse or assistant might spend a few minutes doing this. A final (and more extreme) approach is to ask patients to routinely bring in their medications and count pills. We have not been using pill counts in the office practice, but they are a part of all clinical research trials—on occasion this is *quite* an informative method for detecting noncompliance.

B. Renovascular Hypertension

Renovascular hypertension should be suspected in (1) those individuals with severe hypertension at a very young age (under 25 years); (2) patients in whom severe hypertension develops for the first time at an older age (over 60 years); and (3) patients whose hypertension rapidly worsened although in past years it was previously well controlled on a stable drug regimen (Table 4.3). Patient 1 described above was somewhat unusual in that she developed severe hypertension for the first time at the age of 48, and her renal artery stenosis was secondary to fibromuscular hyperplasia rather than to atherosclerosis. Fibromuscular dysplasia generally develops much earlier in life and leads to stenosis of the vessel by the time an individual is in his or her (mostly women) 20s. Arteries stenosed or occluded secondary to fibromuscular dysplasia are more amenable to revascularization by PTCA than vessels narrowed by heavy atherosclerotic plaque.

The atherosclerotic process occurs in hypertensive patients prematurely; however, typically renal arteries do not become significantly stenotic ($>70\%$) as early in life as coronary arteries do. Thus, we tend to think of the probability of atherosclerotic renovascular hypertension being greater in patients over 60 years old. In hypertensive individuals who smoke cigarettes, it is not uncommon to see overt signs of atherosclerosis a decade earlier. Atherosclerotic renovascular hypertension is often palliated but less frequently totally reversed either by surgical reconstruction or by

Table 4.3 Clinical Features of Renovascular Hypertension

Development of hypertension (severe) at a young age (suspect for fibromuscular dysplasia, especially in white women)

Moderate-to-severe hypertension for the first time in an elderly individual (generally secondary to atherosclerosis)

Acceleration of blood pressure in a previously controlled mild-to-moderate hypertensive

Physical and laboratory signs: abdominal bruit (50%), proteinuria, reduced creatinine clearance, azotemia

Radiographic features: *ultrasound*: unilateral renal size disparity of >2 cm; *renal scan*: unilateral deterioration of renal blood flow and glomerular filtration rate following administration of captopril; *arteriogram*: direct visualization of the stenosis

PTCA. If an individual has been hypertensive for a number of years, the vascular resistance beds are usually permanently abnormal.

An important question that is frequently asked is "What are the best screening tests for renal artery stenosis?" There are two basic issues at hand: First, is there an anatomical lesion present that is hemodynamically significant enough to induce excess secretion of renin? Second, is it likely that correction of this abnormal stenotic area will result in an improved cr normal blood pressure? One test that has become obsolete for the diagnosis of renal artery stenosis is rapid-sequence intravenous pyelography (IVP). The IVP is likely to detect severe cases of renal artery stenosis where the vessel is nearly occluded and ipsilateral renal function is markedly depressed. However, it has a false negative rate in the neighborhood of 25% and, if positive, simply leads to yet another radiological procedure. Renal ultrasound has not been considered a true screening test for renal artery stenosis. However, it is a useful secondary test after the diagnosis has been made by arteriography to detect differences in renal size and to assess whether the kidney is worth saving. Most surgeons will not operate to revascularize a kidney that is under 7 cm in length as its contribution to overall renal function is so minimal.

In the past 2 years, a number of reports have brought about a revival of renal isotope studies by adding a second step to the procedure. Previously, renography could be used to evaluate differences in renal plasma flow and glomerular function with two separate radiotracers (e.g., technetium and DTPA). Subsequently, investigators in several centers in the United States and Europe have demonstrated a marked increase in the sensitivity and specificity of the renogram by performing a second study after administration of the angiotensin-converting enzyme (ACE) inhibitor captopril. In patients with renal artery stenosis, the ACE inhibitors can acutely reduce glomerular function in the kidney with significantly reduced renal blood flow. Thus, a new or worsened functional deficit present on the captopril renogram, which was not present on the first scan, is an indication of the presence of reversible ischemia as well as a good potential for amelioration of the hypertension by some form of revascularization. Both the specificity and sensitivity of the captopril renal scan have been cited to be as high as 95–100%. These screening tests for renovascular hypertension are available to some, but not all, primary care practitioners. When unable to obtain these studies, or when in doubt about the results, it would be perfectly appropriate to refer this type of patient to a specialist in hypertension or nephrology.

C. Primary Aldosteronism

Estimates of the incidence of primary aldosteronism (adrenal adenoma or hyperplasia) in the United States vary from 0.05% to as high as 2%. However, the incidence of primary aldosteronism in an unselected outpatient hypertensive population has been reported to be about 0.7%. Aldosterone overproduction results in elevated blood pressure, hypokalemia and hypomagnesemia, and suppression of the plasma renin activity. Nearly two-thirds of patients with primary aldosteronism have a solitary, semiautonomous adenoma in the adrenal cortex, or Conn's syndrome, while almost all of the rest have idiopathic hyperaldosteronism (usually from bilateral adrenal hyperplasia). Primary aldosteronism is an uncommon cause of resistant hypertension. But in a patient with unexplained hypokalemia and hypertension, a more sophisticated diagnostic evaluation for adrenal adenoma or hyperplasia is needed.

D. Pheochromocytoma

Episodic hypertension may be a sign of adrenergic excess secondary to a pheochromocytoma that secretes either norepinephrine (85–90%), epinephrine (10%), or both (<5%) catecholamine hormones. A minority of patients with pheochromocytoma have sustained hypertension with no history of paroxysms of BP elevation. These patients may fall into a category of resistant hypertension. Thus, it may be reasonable to include a 24-hr collection of urine for catecholamine metabolites (metanephrines and vanillylmandelic acid) in the diagnostic evaluation of a patient with resistant hypertension. Since many antihypertensive agents, especially the alpha- and beta-blockers, interfere with the assay for catecholamine hormones and their metabolites, it is best to perform these studies after tapering the drugs.

E. Office or White-Coat Hypertension

We tend to think of patients with "office" or "white-coat" hypertension as the untreated, mild hypertensives who have a pressor response in the doctor's office and are normotensive in all other situations (see Chapter 1). However, as shown in the case presentation in this chapter, office hypertension can certainly be observed in patients on drug therapy as well. The initial way to screen for the diagnosis of office hypertension is to obtain manual out-of-office BP readings, preferably by the patient. If a large discrepancy between in-office and out-of-office readings is found in an individual in whom there is no clinical evidence of target organ disease, noninvasive, automatic ambulatory BP monitoring should be obtained. In patients who have evidence of serious target organ damage (e.g., proteinuria and abnormal renal function, retinopathy, left ventricular hypertrophy, or peripheral vascular disease), it only makes sense that their long-term BP control has been inadequate. A recent Swedish study by Hartford and colleagues demonstrated that following 7 years of antihypertensive therapy in middle-aged men, target organ involvement from the hypertension (specifically, renal and cardiac function) regressed to a level similar to that of a cohort of age-matched normotensive men. Thus, if long-term antihypertensive therapy has been effective, hemodynamics and target organ abnormalities can return to a normal state.

There are no universally accepted values for ambulatory BP readings, as there are for the office BP. On the other hand, there are a fair amount of data now on normal individuals as well as untreated hypertensives that suggest that an average, awake ambulatory BP of under 135/85 mm Hg and an average, sleeping BP of under 120/80 mm Hg are "normal" or at least associated with

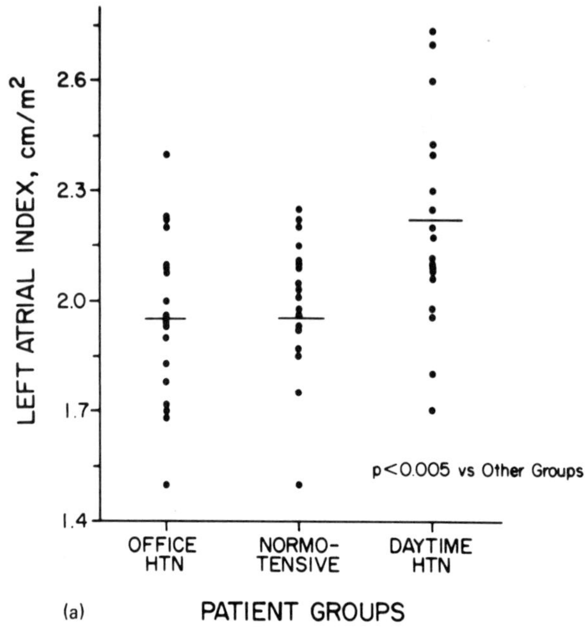

Figure 4.4   Left atrial size, left ventricular mass index, and left ventricular filling rates in patients with office hypertension, normotension, and daytime hypertension. (From White et al., *JAMA*, 1989, 261:873–877.)

a low level of target organ disease. What is lacking in the field of ambulatory BP monitoring is the type of long-term studies that evaluate prognosis as related to the level of ambulatory BP at entry into the trial. Preliminary trials of this type suggest that the ambulatory BP is moderately superior to the office BP in predicting cardiovascular morbidity and mortality. Our group recently assessed never-previously-treated patients for the presence of left ventricular hypertrophy, left atrial abnormalities, and reduced rapid diastolic filling in patients with office hypertension, normotension, and daytime hypertension (elevated BP out-of-office as well as in-office). As shown in Figure 4.4, all three of these cardiac parameters in the office hypertension group were similar to the findings of the normotensive group. These data are further evi-

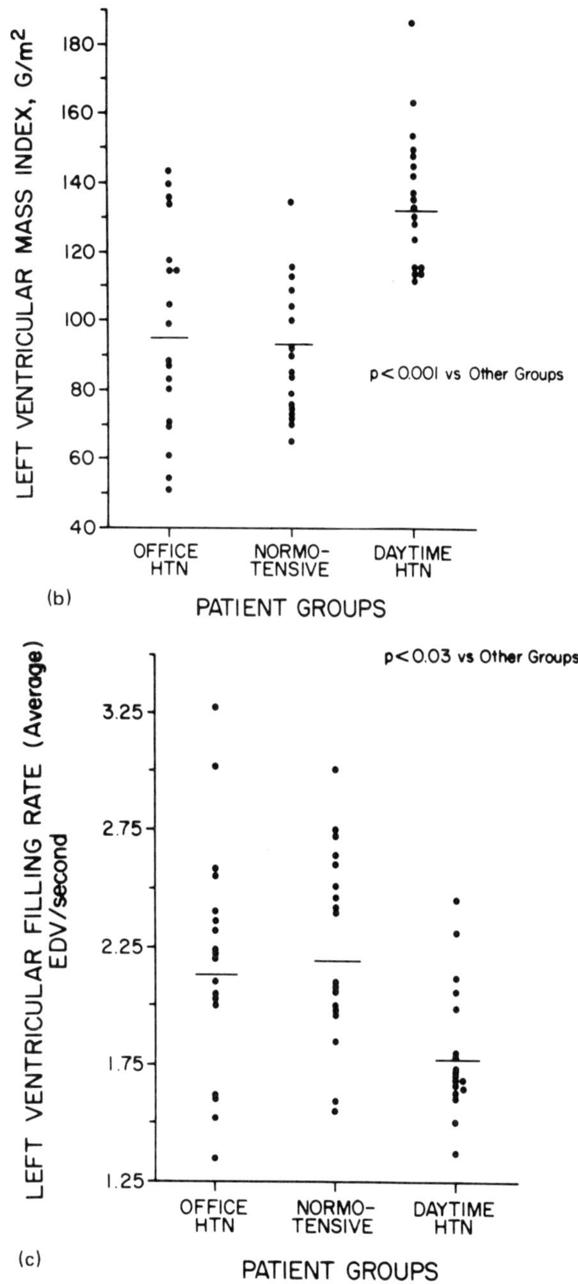

LEFT VENTRICULAR MASS INDEX, G/m²
180
160
140
120
100
80
60
40
p < 0.001 vs Other Groups
OFFICE HTN
NORMO-TENSIVE
DAYTIME HTN
PATIENT GROUPS
(b)
LEFT VENTRICULAR FILLING RATE (Average) EDV/second
p < 0.03 vs Other Groups
3.25
2.75
2.25
1.75
1.25
OFFICE HTN
NORMO-TENSIVE
DAYTIME HTN
PATIENT GROUPS
(c)

dence of the benignity of having an elevated BP only in the doctor's office.

F. Excessive Alcohol Intake and Hypertension

A growing amount of evidence is establishing alcoholism as a secondary cause of hypertension. Sometimes it is difficult to pinpoint the etiology of resistant hypertension to excessive drinking. First, the clinician must think of the diagnosis! Second, one must diplomatically discuss the issue of alcohol abuse and elevated blood pressure with the patient. Recently, we saw a 25-year-old man working as a bank executive who was married to a 4th-year medical student. His referral was the result of her having taken blood pressures at home and finding them to be in the range of 150/100 to 160/110 mm Hg. Indeed, we confirmed these values in the office and found no particular evidence for any usual "secondary" forms of hypertension. When we asked him if he did much drinking or used drugs (e.g., cocaine), he commented that he drank a few beers after dinner on a regular basis, perhaps more on weekends—however, this was nothing new; after all, he had started this practice in college. I suggested that he discontinue the "few beers" on the weekdays completely and hold his weekend drinking to two per day or, better yet, none. Both he and his wife were amazed at the suggestion that his "benign" beer drinking could possibly have anything to do with his hypertension. Four weeks later, following total cessation of alcohol, his home and office BPs averaged 130/80 mm Hg.

Many treated patients drink heavily but then withhold alcohol for 1 or 2 days prior to their visit with the doctor—this leads to a kind of miniwithdrawal, and BP and heart rate are elevated but there are no other signs of alcohol withdrawal. This may also be seen in episodic problem drinkers rather than regular daily consumers of alcohol (e.g., on a Monday afternoon appointment).

Studies from inpatient alcohol programs have reported that as many as 50% of patients entering the hospital have hypertensive readings during the early days of the detoxification program.

The BP returns to normal in the majority of these individuals as long as they abstain from drinking. The suspected cause of BP elevation is excessive catecholamine hormones. In one well-known study, beta-blocker therapy reduced the BP, heart rate, and benzodiazepine requirements in patients going through alcohol withdrawal syndrome.

Thus, if you obtain a history of heavy daily or episodic (e.g., weekend) drinking and have a patient willing to abstain completely for a substantial period of time (either in or out of the hospital), a new reassessment of the hypertension should be performed. If untreated, one might wait a number of weeks, to see whether the BP has become normal, as in the example above. In treated patients, alcohol should be discontinued prior to increasing any doses of the antihypertensive drugs or adding another agent to the regimen.

G.   Drugs, Interactions, and Antagonism

Drug abuse is an uncommon, but potential cause of resistant hypertension. Two types of substance abuse have been observed to cause hypertension, occasionally severely, in our clinics. First is cocaine, which when used regularly, especially through the more potent means, such as smoking "crack" or "freebasing," can cause marked increases in heart rate and blood pressure. Unfortunately, there is no means for detecting this problem other than by history or informed urine screening for cocaine metabolites.

Amphetamine abuse, including over-the-counter stimulants, can also cause hypertension. The sympathomimetic amines (e.g., phenylpropanolamine) should not induce hypertension in low doses, however, when used repeatedly during the day, and in higher doses (> 100 mg phenylpropanolamine or equivalent, daily) they may even induce high BP in a normotensive individual. Over-the-counter diet pills generally contain large quantities of phenylpropanolamine. Numerous cases reported in the literature show accelerated hypertension, myocardial infarction, or intracerebral hemorrhage following ingestion of a few of these tablets by unsuspecting teenagers or foolish adults.

Many over-the-counter decongestants have much less of the vasoactive drug (sympathomimetic amine) than diet pills and would cause little or no problem in a treated hypertensive. Pseudoephedrine and antihistamines have little or no effect on blood pressure. Some of the long-acting, stronger preparations have 50 mg or more of phenylpropanolamine—these should be avoided by hypertensive patients. Many studies now show that doses of 50 mg or more of phenylpropanolamine can induce a transient, but significant rise in blood pressure. Treatment with a beta-adrenergic blocking drug greatly reduces the likelihood of a significant pressor response from a sympathomimetic amine.

As shown in Table 4.4, besides drugs of abuse, a number of prescribed agents can interfere with antihypertensive drugs or can increase the BP by an endogenous mechanism. Oral contraceptives are notable for producing this effect in susceptible women. The most common scenario with oral contraceptives is the young woman who was previously normotensive until the "pill" was started. Following one or two cycles, the BP is mildly or moderately hypertensive and there may be a little pretibial edema. A few weeks after the oral contraceptive is discontinued, the BP returns to normal.

The nonsteroidal antiinflammatory drugs (NSAIDs) have now been shown to attenuate the antihypertensive effects of thiazide diuretics, loop diuretics, beta-adrenergic blockers, alpha-2 agonists, and ACE inhibitors. These drugs reduce the level of the endoge-

Table 4.4   Drugs and Drug Interactions Associated with Resistant Hypertension

Alcohol excess (over 2 oz daily)
Cocaine (especially if ingested through "freebasing")
Amphetamines and "amphetamine-like" drugs (sympathomimetic amines)
Oral contraceptives
Nonsteroidal antiflammatory agents—can attenuate the hypotensive effects of diuretics, ACE inhibitors, sympatholytic drugs
Aspirin—can rarely interfere with actions of ACE inhibitors

nous vasodilators the prostaglandins (particularly, PGE_1 and PGE_2), and thus BP goes up. There may be other mechanisms of drug interference within tissue sites as well. The NSAID sulindac may be an exception to this phenomenon. Aspirin has also been reported to have potential for interference with the effects of the ACE inhibitors.

IV. PRACTICAL ASPECTS OF DRUG THERAPY IN THE RESISTANT HYPERTENSIVE

As mentioned at the beginning of the chapter, patients should be treated with maximally tolerated doses of two or three drugs before being considered resistant to therapy. It is also important to choose antihypertensive drugs that complement each other, e.g., are additive or even synergistic when used together. For example, the thiazide diuretics are additive to ACE inhibitors in patients with moderate or severe hypertension. The diuretics stimulate the renin-angiotensin axis and the ACE inhibitors may be more effective. An example of a lesser combination is the alpha-1 antagonist prazosin together with the alpha-2 agonist clonidine. Clonidine reduces systemic vascular resistance through central mechanisms that inhibit norepinephrine release; the autonomic nervous system is effectively "blunted." Adding a peripherally acting drug such as prazosin has little extra effect when the autonomic nervous system is blocked from a higher level.

Another general principle that is effective in the problem patient is to avoid multiple dosing as much as possible. Most antihypertensive drugs can be given once or twice daily, even if their plasma half-life is 6 or 8 hr. For patients to remember to take pills three or four times daily is difficult and generally impractical. A few years ago, prior to introduction of the longer-acting calcium channel blockers or ACE inhibitors, we performed a study with nifedipine and captopril in combination in a group of 10 resistant hypertensives. We found that several of the patients had loss of effective BP control during the last 2–3 hr of the dosing period even when these drugs were given at 8-hr intervals (Fig. 4.5).

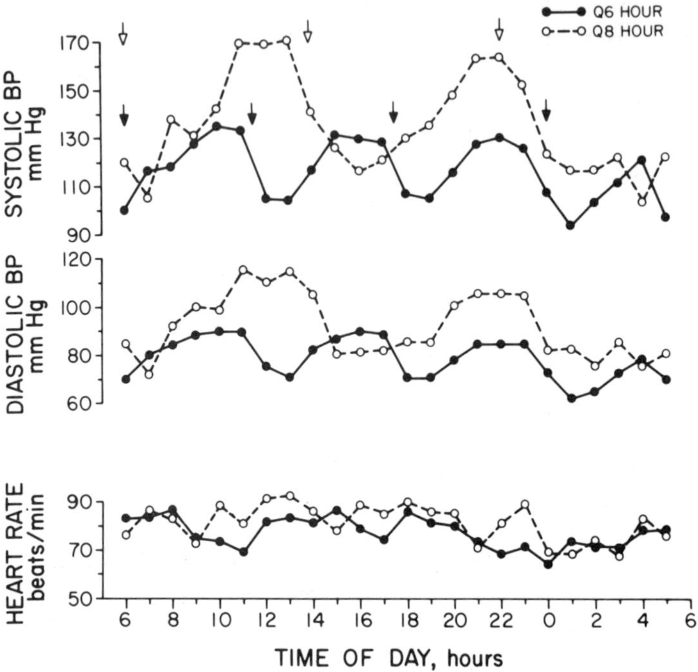

Figure 4.5 Twenty-four-hour curves of blood pressure and heart rate during combined therapy with captopril and nifedipine in a patient with previously resistant hypertension. Arrows show exact time of dosing on a 6-hr (solid symbols) and 8-hr (open symbols) schedule. (From White et al., *Clin Pharmacol Ther*, 1986; 39:43–48, with permission.)

Today, it is possible to use once-daily regimens with the long-acting beta-blockers, diuretics, verapamil-SR, ACE inhibitors, and even minoxidil. However, some of the agents that are effective when given once daily in mild-to-moderate hypertensives (e.g., verapamil-SR, enalapril, nitrendipine) should be given twice daily to maintain good BP control in a severe or resistant hypertensive patient. In patients who have resistant hypertension secondary to poor malabsorption due to gastric or intestinal disease, possibly with bypass surgery, we have used transdermal clonidine with great success. The drug is delivered through the skin for 7 days and

Table 4.5   General Principles of Drug Therapy in Resistant Hypertension

Use combinations that are additive or synergistic
Use long-acting preparations to provide once- or twice-daily dosing
Specific combinations with proven benefit:
   ACE inhibitors and diuretics—may cause deterioration in renal function
   ACE inhibitors and calcium channel blockers—potent vasodilation is effective in broad variety of patients
   ACE inhibitors and alpha-beta blockers—potent vasodilation but postural hypotension can be problematic
   Beta blockers and calcium channel blockers (especially dihydropyridine calcium channel blockers)
   Diuretic, long-acting beta-blockers, minoxidil
   Transdermal clonidine—particularly useful when gastrointestinal absorption is impaired

eliminates the need for numerous other agents or frequent dosing. Transdermal clonidine may also be useful in improving compliance and BP control in patients who have problems remembering to take second or multiple doses of oral preparations. (See Table 4.5.)

A number of hypertension specialists have had extensive experience with the direct vasodilator minoxidil. This drug will often work in patients when no other agent is effective, especially in patients with renal failure. However, its side effect profile is not very good and includes hypertrichosis, reflex tachycardia, and volume retention. Minoxidil must be used in combination with a loop diuretic and a beta-adrenergic blocking agent. The drug should be used with caution in patients with underlying coronary disease since even in individuals on beta-blockers the cardiac output is increased by 50–100% following its administration.

REFERENCES

Gifford R W. An algorithm for the management of resistant hypertension. *Hypertension* 1988 11:(Suppl II):101–105.

Hartford M, Wendelhag I, Berglund G, et al. Cardiovascular and renal effects of long-term antihypertensive treatment. *JAMA* 1988;259:2553-2557.

Johns D W, Peack M. Factors that contribute to resistant forms of hypertension: Pharmacological considerations. *Hypertension* 11 1988 (Suppl II): 88-95.

Melby J C. Primary aldosteronism. *Kidney Int* 1984;26:769--778.

Pentel P. Toxicity of over-the-counter stimulants. *JAMA* 1984; 252:1898-1903.

Saunders J B, Beevers D G, Paton A. Alcohol-induced hypertension. *Lancet* 1981;2:653-656.

White W B. Management of resistant hypertension. *Emergency Decisions* 1988;4:7-13.

White W B, Viadero J J, Lane T J, Podesla S. Effects of combination therapy with captopril and nifedipine in severe or resistant hypertension. *Clin Pharmacol Ther* 1986;39:43-48.

White W B, Schulman P, McCabe E J, Dey H M. Average daily blood pressure not office blood pressure predicts cardiac function in patients with hypertension. *JAMA* 1989;261:873-877.

5

The Hypertensive Patient with Coronary Heart Disease

I. ILLUSTRATIVE CASE

A 59-year-old man presented to the emergency room following the onset of chest pain associated with mild lightheadedness and nausea while raking his lawn in October 1988. He was pain-free by the time he arrived at the emergency room. Prior to this episode of pain, he occasionally had had some mild shortness of breath with exertion.

On examination, his weight was 185 lb, heart rate was 86 beats/min (bpm), and blood pressure (BP) was 170/105 mm Hg. There was no retinopathy, and examination of the peripheral vessels was normal. On cardiac examination, a 4th heart sound was auscultated. The remainder of the physical examination was normal.

The electrocardiogram showed a sinus rhythm at 84 bpm, with normal conduction times. The axis was $-35°$ and a left atrial abnormality was present. The R waves in V_{4-6} were 15 mm and the S wave in V_{1-2} was 12 mm; the ST segments and T waves were normal. No ectopic beats were noted. There was no evidence of acute ischemia or infarction. The cardiac enzymes were normal.

The patient was admitted to the coronary care unit for observation for new-onset angina pectoris. Serial cardiac enzymes and electrocardiograms showed no changes over the next 36 hr. The chest pain never did recur while the patient was in the hospital. The heart rate ranged from 72 to 88 bpm and the blood pressure from 130/90 to 160/110 mm Hg. A modified Bruce protocol was performed on the morning of the 3rd hospital day. The patient developed chest tightness following 6 min of exercise at 2.4 mph and 10% grade. Associated with the chest pain was 1 mm depression of the ST segments in V_{3-6} with no changes in the T wave. The ST-segment abnormalities disappeared at the end of the first minute of recovery. Systolic blood pressure peaked at 210 mm Hg while the heart rate rose to 135 bpm during stage 2 of the study.

Two-D echocardiography showed normal wall motion. The left atrial dimension was 4.5 cm (normal, <4.0 cm). Mild left ventricular hypertrophy was present. A radioisotope study demonstrated a resting ejection fraction of 55% (normal >50%), which increased to 57% with exercise. The peak filling rate during diastole was 1.75 end-diastolic volumes/sec (normal >2.0 end-diastolic volumes/sec). There was mild apical hypokinesis during peak exercise, but otherwise the study was normal.

Coronary angiography was recommended to the patient to rule out disease that might be amenable to coronary artery surgery or angioplasty. However, the patient refused the procedure. The physician decided that the best initial treatment for both the coronary artery disease and moderate hypertension was beta-adrenergic blockers plus long-acting nitrates. Thus, the patient was started on metoprolol, 50 mg twice daily, and long-acting isorbide dinitrate, 40 mg twice daily. On discharge from the hospital, the heart rate was 64 bpm and the resting, seated BP was 132/84 mm Hg.

An exercise treadmill test was repeated 2 weeks following hospital discharge. The patient walked for 9 min and did not develop chest pain. No electrocardiographic abnormalities were observed. Follow-up over the next year demonstrated good blood pressure control and no further chest pain.

A. Comments

While it has typically been a point of controversy, the majority of cardiologists would have recommended that this patient undergo coronary arteriography. In any event, he was found to have hypertension that required a new antihypertensive regimen. The calcium channel blockers are an alternative initial therapy to the beta-blockers in a patient like the one described here. If his exercise treadmill test had induced chest pain or electrocardiographic abnormalities, or if he had sustained chest pain on the treatment regimen, coronary arteriography would have been even more strongly advised. The nitrates may be used in combination with all antianginal, antihypertensive regimens and clearly are beneficial for ischemia. However, their efficacy in lowering blood pressure is unpredictable.

II. PATHOPHYSIOLOGICAL CONSIDERATIONS

The association between hypertension and coronary artery disease is partly explained by the effects of increased arterial wall tension on the vascular smooth muscle. The wall of the artery hypertrophies and the lumen narrows. Where there is vessel damage (associated with this smooth muscle hyperplasia), the greatest possibility exists for the atherosclerotic process to occur.

The basic abnormality that is produced by occlusive arterial disease, whether secondary to hypertension or to the other cardiac risk factors, is tissue ischemia. Stenoses of over 75% can induce impairment of resting flow to the myocardium, but lesser stenoses may cause problems during exercise when myocardial demands are greater. The level of systemic arterial pressure is also important when coronary artery disease is present. If the BP is high, the compliance of the ventricle is reduced, and this may cause left ventricular dysfunction. In contrast, if the BP is too low, coronary flow may be impaired, and epicardial ischemia may worsen.

III. LEFT VENTRICULAR HYPERTROPHY

One of the major independent risk factors associated with the development of ischemic heart disease, congestive heart failure, and sudden death in hypertensive patients is left ventricular enlargement or hypertrophy (LVH). In past years, the electrocardiogram (ECG) has been used to identify the presence of LVH and has significantly underestimated its prevalence. The echocardiogram, on the other hand, has been shown to be much more sensitive than the ECG in detecting LVH. When evaluated by M-mode echocardiography, the estimated incidence of LVH in untreated mildly to moderately hypertensive patients exceeds 60%. In the same group of individuals, the ECG may show criteria for LVH in only 10%. The presence of LVH by ECG has been associated with a number of morbid conditions (Table 5.1), including an increased incidence of ventricular ectopy, myocardial infarction, and death. Prospective, long-term studies of a similar nature using the echocardiogram for the diagnosis of LVH are under way at the present time.

Radionuclide ventriculography (gated blood pool scans) shows abnormalities in left ventricular diastolic filling in patients with hypertension (Fig. 5.1a), occasionally even before there is

Table 5.1   Problems Associated with Left Ventricular Hypertrophy

Impaired diastolic filling time
Increase in ventricular ectopy (including ventricular tachycardia)
Congestive heart failure
Ischemic heart disease (functional)
Sudden death

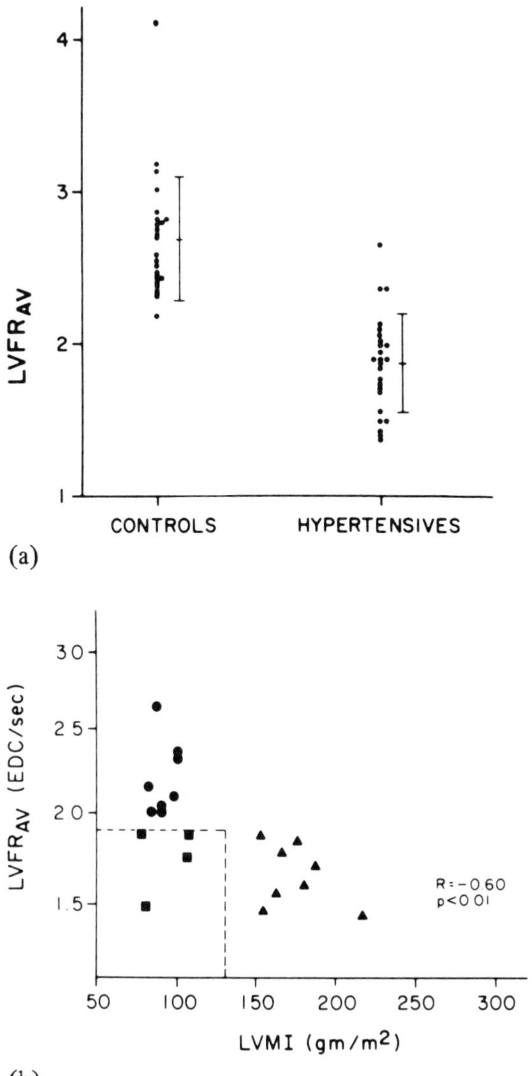

Figure 5.1 (a) Left ventricular filling rate is depressed in mild-to-moderate hypertensives compared to normotensive, age-matched controls. (b) Relationship between left ventricular filling and left ventricular mass index in hypertensive patients. The dashed horizontal line represents the lower level of normal filling rate while the dashed vertical line represents the upper limits of normal of left ventricular mass index. The squares are subjects with normal mass but reduced filling rates. (From Smith VE et al., *J Am Coll Cardiol* 1985; 5:869–874, with permission.)

echocardiographically defined hypertrophy and nearly always prior to any abnormalities in systolic ejection function (Fig. 5.1b). In hypertensive patients with very mild LVH, these filling abnormalities do not appear to induce any symptoms. However, in longstanding LVH, the impairment of pumping function of the heart can lead to congestive heart failure. When coronary atherosclerosis is also present, LVH exacerbates myocardial ischemia and worsens the symptoms of angina pectoris.

A. Regression of Left Ventricular Hypertrophy

Left ventricular hypertrophy may be reversed (or its development delayed) by antihypertensive drug therapy. In consideration of the many deleterious effects associated with LVH, an ability to induce regression of LVH has become an important attribute for antihypertensive agents since such an effect may provide cardioprotection. There are preliminary data from the Framingham study that show that regression of LVH (ECG, not echocardiographic) is associated with less mortality and cardiovascular morbidity than in hypertensive patients who did not show regression of LVH by ECG. Thus, antihypertensive agents that prevent progression of hypertrophy are favored over the drugs that either do not effect LVH or stimulate an increase in myocardial mass.

Regression of left ventricular mass in hypertensive patients occurs following treatment with many classes of antihypertensive drugs. While effectively lowering BP, the thiazide diuretics (Fig. 5.2) are one class of antihypertensives that do *not* seem to induce a change in left ventricular mass or wall thickness. Direct vasodilators, such as hydralazine or minoxidil, have also been reported to bring about either no change in or even increase in the left ventricular mass in patients with hypertension. Most studies evaluating ACE inhibitors, alpha-2 agonists, alpha-1 antagonists, beta-adrenergic blocking drugs, and some of the calcium channel blockers have demonstrated regression of LVH in hypertensive patients. Unfortunately, many of the LVH regression studies performed in the last few years had major flaws in either methodology or study design. For example, what is a significant regression in left ventric-

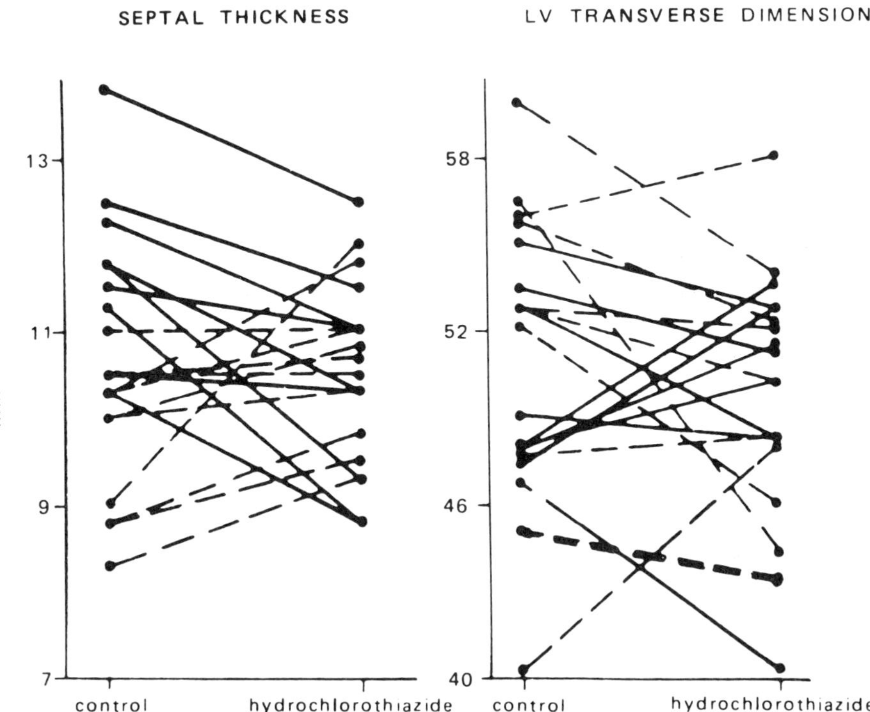

Figure 5.2 Changes in ventricular septal thickness (left) and left ventricular transverse dimension (right) following 6 weeks of hydrochlorothiazide treatment (100 mg/day) in hypertensive patients. There was no net change in the group despite significant lowering of BP. (From Drayer et al., *Clin Pharmacol Ther* 1982; 32:283-288, with permission.)

ular mass index? If one is to use a statistical test and there are more than 20 patients in the study, a 4% reduction in mass could easily become statistically significant. We now realize that the observer error for the determination of left ventricular mass by highly trained and experienced echocardiographers is about 5%—so a 4% reduction could be associated with observer error, rather than a drug effect.

In the past 2 years, clinical studies have shown that some classes of antihypertensive drugs regress LVH while simultaneously improving cardiac function. One such study that we performed in Connecticut showed that about a 15% improvement in diastolic function occurred in previously untreated hypertensive patients with LVH following therapy with the beta-blocker metoprolol (Fig. 5.3). While not all patients had regression of the left ventricular mass, nearly all of them had improvement in diastolic function. It is known that functional abnormalities may occur before structural changes, and now there is evidence that these physiological changes can be reverted toward normal with antihypertensive drug therapy. Similar findings to our data with metoprolol have also been reported with the angiotensin-converting enzyme inhibitors and some of the calcium channel blockers.

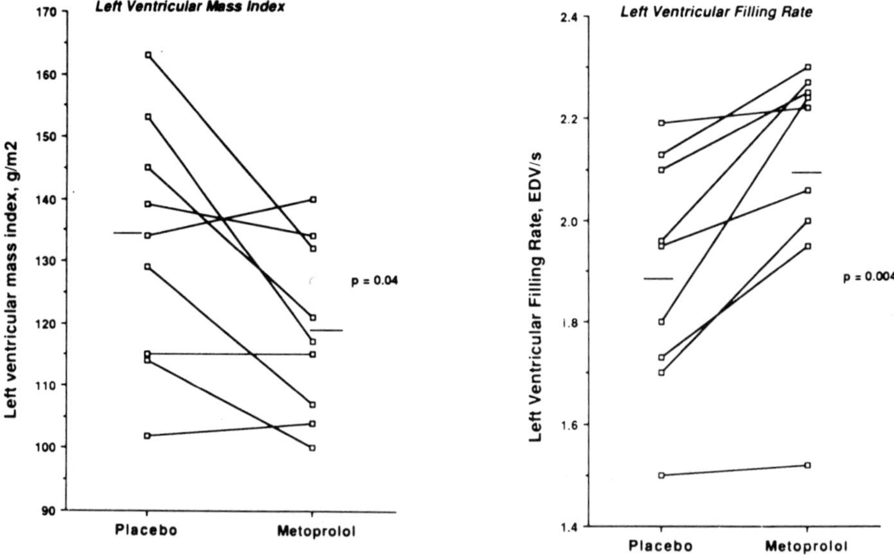

Figure 5.3   Individual effects of metoprolol therapy for 6 months on left ventricular mass index (left) and rapid, left ventricular filling rate (right) in patients with mild-to-moderate hypertension. (From White et al., *Am Heart J* 1989; 117:145–152, with permission.)

IV. CONSIDERATIONS FOR ANTIHYPERTENSIVE DRUG THERAPY IN PATIENTS WITH CORONARY HEART DISEASE

Lowering elevated blood pressure can decrease the severity of angina pectoris; therefore, careful consideration should be given to selecting antihypertensive therapy in patients with both concomitant hypertension and coronary heart disease. An ideal agent for the treatment of hypertension complicated by symptomatic coronary artery disease should have a number of particular characteristics (Table 5.2). The drug should also be an effective antianginal agent and should be able to reduce blood pressure at rest as well as during exertion. It is advantageous if the agent produces little or no reflex stimulation of the sympathetic nervous system. A vasodilator like hydralazine can possibly precipitate angina pectoris by causing reflex tachycardia and increasing myocardial oxygen demand. Another problem with the direct vasodilators is that they can induce a "steal" syndrome, where myocardial perfusion pressure distal to a coronary artery stenosis is reduced by dilatation of small arterioles.

In the arrhythmia-prone patient with hypertension, the arrhythmogenic (or antiarrhythmogenic) potential of a drug is an important consideration. The thiazide and loop diuretics, which are frequently used as antihypertensive agents in patient with coronary disease, can induce hypomagnesemia and hypokalemia, which has been associated with serious ventricular arrhythmias.

Table 5.2 Advantageous Features of Agents Used in Both the Management of Hypertension and Angina Pectoris

---

Improves coronary blood flow while lowering blood pressure
No expansion of the intravascular volume
Lack of development of tolerance
Desirable effect on other risk factors (e.g., lipids, blood glucose) to prevent the progression of the atherosclerotic process
Minimal adverse effects on common comorbid illnesses (chronic lung disease, peripheral vascular disease, diabetes mellitus)

The diuretics do not appear to cause much change in ventricular irritability in uncomplicated hypertensive patients even when inducing mild hypokalemia. However, the concern for increasing the frequency of ventricular extrasystoles by drug-induced hypokalemia is accelerated when almost any ECG abnormality is present, including left ventricular hypertrophy. Thus, proper potassium replacement or potassium-sparing diuretics should be administered when diuretics are used in hypertensive patients with underlying ischemic heart disease. Maintenance of a normal plasma potassium is especially important in patients receiving cardiac glycosides, in view of the ability of hypokalemia to exacerbate digitalis toxicity.

Patients with hypertension and coronary heart disease or those who are at substantial risk for the development of ischemic heart disease should be treated with drugs that improve both conditions. Pharmacological agents, such as the thiazide diuretics, that impact adversely on other cardiovascular risk factors (including hypercholesterolemia, hyperglycemia, and hyperuricemia) are not ideal for initial therapy of hypertension in the presence of coronary artery disease. Other agents that also have modestly negative impact on lipids, e.g., nonselective beta-blocking drugs, markedly benefit patients with coronary artery disease. Thus, the latter agents are considered appropriate for the initial management of hypertension in the face of ischemic heart disease. (A more complete discussion of the adverse metabolic effects of antihypertensive drugs can be found in Chapter 7.)

V. SPECIFIC THERAPY FOR HYPERTENSIVE PATIENTS WITH CORONARY HEART DISEASE

A. Beta-adrenergic Blocking Agents

The beta-blocking drugs were actually used for the treatment of angina pectoris prior to their use in hypertension. These drugs inhibit catecholamine binding to beta-receptors, thus reducing endogenous catecholamine-induced increments in BP, heart rate, and contractility of the myocardium. The beta-blocking drugs improve the balance between coronary blood flow (*supply*) and myocardial oxygen consumption (*demand*) in patients with stenotic coronary arteries.

The beta-1 receptors in the heart mediate increases in both the heart rate and inotropy and are blocked by both beta-1-selective and nonselective beta-blockers (Table 5.3). The beta-blockers with intrinsic sympathomimetic activity (ISA, also called partial agonist activity) have little effect on the heart rate at rest and are not recommended for patients with angina pectoris at rest. Furthermore, ISA-containing beta-blockers should probably be avoided in patients with angina and a low heart rate since these agents may actually exacerbate angina by increasing heart rate. Another situation that deserves caution is when making a transition from a non-ISA-containing beta-blocker to an ISA-containing beta-blocker in a hypertensive patient with coronary disease. We have observed patients develop worsened angina within a few days of the changeover to the ISA-containing beta-blocker.

Table 5.3   The Beta-blocking Agents (Clinically Available in the United States)

Agent	Receptor selectivity	ISA-containing	Usual dose for hypertension
Acebutolol	Beta-1	Yes	400–800 mg q.d.
Atenolol	Beta-1	No	25–100 mg q.d.
Labetalol	Beta-1, -2, and alpha-1	Yes (beta-2)	100–600 mg b.i.d.
Metoprolol	Beta-1	No	25–200 mg b.i.d.[a]
Nadolol	Beta-1, -2	No	20–160 mg q.d.
Penbutolol	Beta-1, -2	Yes	20–40 mg q.d.
Pindolol	Beta-1, -2	Yes	5–30 mg b.i.d.
Propranolol	Beta-1, -2	No	20–160 mg b.i.d.
Propranolol-LA	Beta-1, -2	No	60–160 mg q.d.
Timolol	Beta-1, -2	No	5–20 mg t.i.d.

Always start with the lowest available dose.

q.d., once daily; b.i.d., twice daily; t.i.d., thrice daily.

[a]Metoprolol can also be administered once daily for hypertension. Atenolol, metoprolol, nadolol, propranolol, and timolol are approved for the treatment of angina pectoris.

An important aspect of care of the patient with coronary heart disease is *secondary prevention* of myocardial infarction. A large number of well-done clinical trials have demonstrated that non-ISA beta-blocking agents reduce reinfarction following acute myocardial infarction. Over periods of 1–6 years, the average reduction in mortality in patients treated with a beta-blocker (versus placebo) is between 25 and 35%. In many of the beta-adrenergic blocking agent trials following acute myocardial infarction, reductions in sudden death, nonfatal reinfarction, and other manifestations of cardiac ischemia, including ventricular arrhythmias, were observed. The most important mechanisms by which the beta-blocking agents prevent reinfarction or reduce the severity of the infarction include reduction in cardiac oxygen demand, catecholamine-induced rapid arrhythmias, and myocardial metabolic effects.

Thus, all hypertensive patients who have had a recent acute myocardial infarction should be considered candidates for beta-adrenergic blocking agents unless there are fairly strong contraindications to beta-blockade (Table 5.4). The modest negative effect that the non-ISA-containing beta-blockers have on lipids is outweighed by the beneficial data that demonstrate cardioprotection for a few years following a myocardial infarction.

The abrupt discontinuation of a beta-blocking agent in a patient with hypertension and coronary artery disease can lead to a marked increase in heart rate and blood pressure. Not infrequently, this can exacerbate symptoms of angina pectoris and cause myocardial infarction and even death. Thus, one must always at-

Table 5.4 Contraindications for the Use of Beta-blocking Agents

Bronchial asthma (including with ISA-containing drugs)
Severe left ventricular dysfunction with CHF
Second- or third-degree atrioventricular block
Sinus bradycardia (<50 bpm)
Severe hepatic impairment
Unstable type I diabetes mellitus

tempt to taper a beta-blocker to a very small dose before discontinuing the drug entirely. There are data to suggest that the "withdrawal" syndrome with beta-blockers is more intense with drugs that have short plasma half-lives (propranolol, timolol). However, I have occasionally observed patients develop beta-blocker withdrawal syndrome with some of the longer-acting agents as well. Finally, the combination of an alpha-2 agonist and beta-blocking drug should probably be avoided in patients with hypertension and coronary heart disease. Abrupt cessation of the alpha-2 agonist leads to marked increase in unopposed alpha-mediated vasoconstriction (because the beta-blocker is inhibiting beta-2 receptors that mediate vasodilation) and severe hypertension.

B. Calcium Channel Blockers

The calcium channel blockers inhibit vasoconstriction in coronary and peripheral arterial smooth muscle. Individual drugs within this class of antihypertensives have variable effects on the heart with regard to myocardial contractility, chronotropy, and conduction in the AV node. The dihydropyridine calcium channel blockers (e.g., nifedipine, nitrendipine, and nicardipine) are more potent inhibitors of the calcium channels in vascular smooth muscle than in the heart. Diltiazem and verapamil are approximately equal in potency in the heart and vascular smooth muscle.

All the currently available calcium channel blocking agents (Table 5.5) have been shown to reduce the frequency of angina pectoris. Furthermore, these agents improve exercise tolerance in patients with chronic stable angina, lower systemic arterial pressure, and prevent recurrence of myocardial ischemia at rest. All calcium channel blockers lower systemic vascular resistance, but verapamil and diltiazem also slow heart rate and modestly reduce myocardial contractility. Of particular importance for patients with angina pectoris is that calcium channel blockers directly increase coronary blood flow.

In the past few years, a number of new calcium channel blockers, differing in pharmacological activity, have been intro-

Table 5.5 The Calcium Channel Blocking Agents (Different Formulations)

Name	Vasodilator effects	Myocardial effects	Usual dosages
Diltiazem	++	++	30–180 mg t.i.d.
Diltiazem-SR	++	++	60–180 mg b.i.d.
Felodipine-ER	+++	+	2.5–10 mg q.d.
Nicardipine	+++	+	10–30 mg t.i.d.
Nicardipine-SR	+++	+	10–30 mg b.i.d.
Nifedipine	+++	+	10–30 mg q.i.d.
Nifedipine-SR	+++	+	20–100 mg q.d.
Nifedipine-GITS	+++	+	30–120 mg q.d.
Nitrendipine	+++	+	5–20 mg b.i.d.
Verapamil	+	+++	40–160 mg b.i.d.
Verapamil-SR	+	+++	120–480 mg q.d.

Always start with the lowest recommended dose.
SR, sustained release; ER, extended release; GITS, gastrointestinal transport system.

duced (Table 5.5). However, there are not very marked differences in effects on BP and angina among the different dihydropyridines. Individual patients may find one agent has less vasodilator side effects than another, but no generalizations can be made except that the longer-acting calcium channel blockers have a less abrupt onset of action and cause less facial flushing, palpitations, and vasodilator-type headaches. With long-term administration (>2 weeks), most, if not all, of these "vasodilator" side effects associated with the calcium channel blockers disappear. Pretibial edema, which is secondary to dilation of small venules in dependent areas and not volume retention with weight gain, can be a persistent problem in approximately 5–10% of patients taking calcium channel blockers. Constipation appears to be an adverse side effect relatively unique to verapamil or verapamil-SR. If the drug is beneficial and a decision is made to maintain the verapamil, psyllium seed preparations (e.g., metamucil) seem to counteract the problem quite effectively.

A number of clinical studies have now been performed with diltiazam, nicardipine, nifedipine, nitrendipine, and verapamil in patients with both angina pectoris and hypertension. There are comparable effects by these drugs to reduce angina frequency and nitroglycerin consumption and improve exercise tolerance. Diltiazem and verapamil lower resting heart rate more than nicardipine, nifedipine or nitrendipine. The beneficial antianginal effects of the calcium channel blockers can be explained by the ability of these drugs to improve coronary blood flow and reduce the rate-pressure product during exertion.

Compared to the beta-adrenergic blocking agents, the calcium channel blockers do not fare as well with regard to secondary prevention of myocardial infarction. In studies of nifedipine and verapamil versus a placebo group, neither mortality nor size of infarct was improved following therapy with those calcium channel blockers in patients who had sustained a myocardial infarction. A recent secondary prevention study with diltiazem (Diltiazem Post-Infarction Trial, DPIT) demonstrated disparate effects following 1–3 years of follow-up, depending on the functional status of the left ventricle (Fig. 5.4). In patients with normal left ventricular function, diltiazem appeared to significantly reduce post-myocardial infarction morbidity/mortality, whereas in those patients with pulmonary vascular congestion at the time of the acute infarction, the long-term outcome was worse on diltiazem than placebo. The reason for this remarkable finding remains to be elucidated.

C. Combination Therapy

The calcium channel blockers can be combined with the beta-blocking agents when one agent is unsuccessful in maintaining control of BP or angina attacks. It is relatively common practice to combine a calcium channel blocker of the dihydropyridine type (nifedipine, nitrendipine, nicardipine) with a beta-blocker. Diltiazem and verapamil can be combined with a beta-blocker, but caution must be exercised since either calcium channel blocker can prolong AV conduction or induce a bradycardia; thus, combining

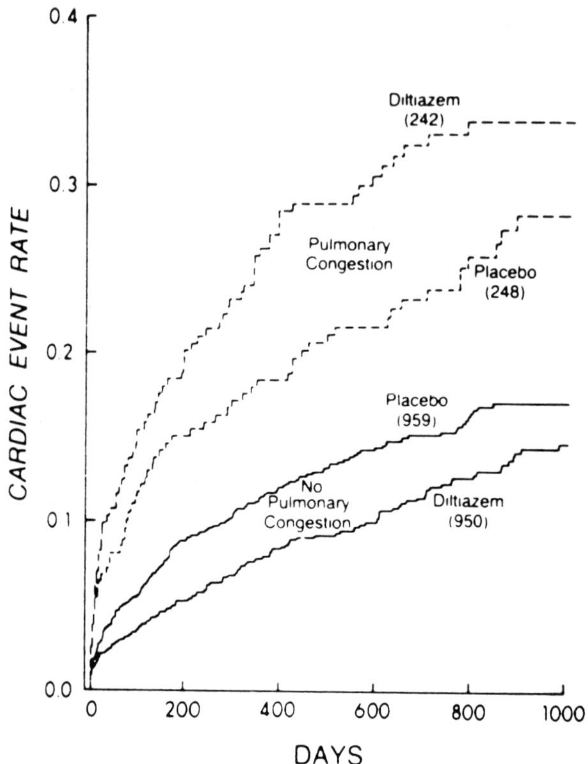

Figure 5.4 Effects of the calcium channel blocker diltiazem versus placebo on cardiac events in patients with recent myocardial infarction (MI). Patients with normal left ventricular function at the time of the acute MI had better outcomes on diltiazem while those with abnormal left ventricular function had worse outcome on diltiazem than placebo. (From the Multicenter DPIT, *N Engl J Med* 1988; 319:385–392, with permission.)

either verapamil or diltiazem with a beta-blocker may cause a first-degree AV block to become a second-degree AV block or may convert a sinus bradycardia into a junctional bradycardia.

The ACE inhibitors can also be combined with beta-blockers or calcium channel blockers in patients with angina and hypertension. Details regarding the ACE inhibitors are given in the next chapter.

D. Long-Acting Nitrates in Combination with Antihypertensive, Antianginal Drugs

A number of studies have demonstrated that adding a long-acting nitrate to a calcium channel blocker or a beta-blocking agent produces a greater therapeutic effect than single-drug therapy in most patients with angina pectoris. Combining a long-acting nitrate with a calcium channel blocker or beta-blocker should be initiated to reduce myocardial ischemia, and not to further reduce BP. The long-acting nitrates do reduce preload, but do not have predictable effects on systemic arterial pressure. If BP is elevated secondary to chest pain, then it is likely that nitroglycerin preparations will lower the BP since the pain and adrenergic stimuli associated with the pain are removed. During long-term administration, the nitrates may not lower BP at all. On the other hand, occasionally when nitrates and calcium channel blockers are first combined, reduced preload and systemic vascular resistance may result in severe postural hypotension. If the dose of the first vasodilator is reduced slightly just before the second one is added, hypotension is less likely to occur.

REFERENCES

Beta-blocker Heart Attack Trial Research Group. A randomized trial of propranolol in patients with acute myocardial infarction. I. Mortality results. *JAMA* 1982; 247:1707-1714.

Danish Study Group on Verapamil in Myocardial Infarction. Verapamil in acute myocardial infarction. *Eur Heart J* 1984; 5:516-528.

Drayer J I M, Gardin J M, Weber M A, Aronow W S. Changes in ventricular septal thickness during diuretic therapy. *Clin Pharmacol Ther* 1982; 92:283-288.

Hjalmarson A, Elmfeldt D, Herlitz J, et al. Effects of mortality of metoprolol in acute myocardial infarction: A double-blind randomized trial. *Lancet* 1981; 2:823-827.

Muller J E, Morrison J, Stone P H, et al. Nifedipine therapy for patients with threatened and acute myocardial infarction: A randomized, double-blind, placebo-controlled comparison. *Circulation* 1984; 69:740-747.

Multicenter Diltiazem Post-infarction Trial Research Group. The effect of diltiazem on mortality and reinfarction after myocardial infarction. *N Engl J Med* 1988; 319:385-392.

O'Rourke R A. Rationale for calcium entry-blocking drugs in systemic hypertension complicated by coronary artery disease. *Am J Cardiol* 1985; 56:34H-40H.

Smith V E, Schulman P, Karimeddini M K, White W B, Meeran M K, Katz A M. Rapid left ventricular filling in left ventricular hypertrophy: II. Pathologic hypertrophy. *J Am Coll Cardiol* 1985; 5:869-874.

Smith V E, White W B, Meeran M K, Karimeddini M K. Improved left ventricular filling accompanies reduced left ventricular mass during therapy of essential hypertension. *J Am Coll Cardiol* 1986; 8:1449-1454.

White W B, Schulman P, Karimeddini M K, Smith V E. Regression of left ventricular mass is accompanied by improvement in rapid left ventricular filling following antihypertensive therapy with metoprolol. *Am Heart J* 1989; 117:145-152.

6

Management of Hypertension in the Presence of Congestive Heart Failure

In the previous chapter, the problem of hypertension coexisting with coronary heart disease, specifically angina pectoris or myocardial infarction, was discussed. Patients with coronary heart disease and hypertension have another common cardiac manifestation of their underlying pathology in the form of left ventricular dysfunction. The management of congestive heart failure (CHF) has changed considerably in the last few years, thus creating the need for this brief chapter focusing on the new therapeutic regimens that are recommended for patients with concomitant hypertension and CHF.

I. ILLUSTRATIVE CASE

In 1984, a 68-year-old retired college professor presented to the hypertension unit with moderate hypertension. He had been hospitalized the month before to have a myelogram for suspected lumbar disc disease. During the hospitalization, his blood pressure (BP) was moderately to severely elevated (160/110 to 180/120 mm Hg) despite hydrochlorothiazide, 25 mg daily, propranolol, 80 mg b.i.d., and prazosin, 2 mg b.i.d. It soon became apparent that the patient had been abusing alcohol, as he developed sinus tachycardia, tremulousness, and mild emotional lability 12–18 hr following admission to the hospital. This was treated without much difficulty with the benzodiazepine oxazepam. His antihypertensive drug regimen was subsequently altered to hydrochlorothiazide, pindolol, 30 mg b.i.d. (when the propranolol dose was increased, the patient developed a marked sinus bradycardia), and prazosin, 4 mg b.i.d., with BPs ranging from 140/80 to 150/95 mm Hg. Laboratory examination during the hospitalization revealed mild renal insufficiency (serum creatinine 1.6 mg/dl and blood urea nitrogen 23 mg/dl), liver enzymes elevated to twice the normal values, and left ventricular hypertrophy by electrocardiogram.

At outpatient follow-up visit, the BP was in the range of 160/95 to 165/100 mm Hg. The prazosin was increased to 8 mg b.i.d. and subsequent readings were approximately 140/80 mm Hg. The renal function was stable and the patient discontinued drinking alcohol following a 21-day detoxification program.

In October 1985, the patient began to note shortness of breath on exertion, mostly when taking his dog for a stroll, but occasionally just with the minimal exertion associated with walking the 200-ft driveway to the mailbox. The shortness of breath was never accompanied by chest pain or lightheadedness. In November 1985, mild swelling of his ankles and feet was occurring at the end of the day; however, it was not usually present upon awakening.

On physical examination in November 1985, the BP was 160/98 mm Hg with a heart rate of 78 bpm. The jugular veins were not distended at 45°. Examination of the chest demonstrated fine rales at both bases which did not clear upon coughing. On examination of the heart there was a 4th heart sound, and a short midsystolic murmur heard best at the cardiac apex. A 3rd heart sound was not present. The liver edge was palpated 2–3 cm below the right subcostal margin (but this was an old physical finding). Mild pretibial and presacral edema were present. Laboratory studies showed normal serum electrolytes, a serum creatinine of 1.5 mg/dl, and blood urea nitrogen of 22 mg/dl. The electrocardiogram showed a sinus rhythm of 76 bpm, normal P-R and QRS intervals, an axis of $-40°$, and left ventricular hypertrophy (left atrial abnormality, and 50 mm of voltage by adding the R wave in V_5 and the S wave in V_1). No ischemic changes were present. Echocardiography again demonstrated the left ventricular hypertrophy but no dilatation of the ventricular chambers. Radionuclide ventriculography showed a resting left ventricular ejection fraction of 42% (normal $> 55\%$) and a diastolic filling rate of 1.60 end-diastolic volumes (edv) per second (normal > 1.9 edv/second). During supine bicycle exercise, the systolic BP increased to 220 mm Hg, heart rate to 128 bpm, but the ejection fraction remained at 42%. No wall motion abnormalities were observed during exercise.

Since the patient's symptoms were relatively mild, and there was modest renal insufficiency, the diuretic was switched from the thiazide to furosemide, 20 mg b.i.d. Within 48 hr, the patient noted a major improvement. His edema had resolved and he was no longer short of breath when he went to get his newspaper or mail. On reexamination the next week, the BP was 135/85 mm Hg, heart rate 70 bpm, and the lung fields were clear. Serum potassium had dropped to 3.4 mEq/liter (from 3.9 mEq/liter) but all the other serum chemistries were stable. The patient started potassium supplementation (40 mEq daily) and was advised to follow a diet high in potassium and low in sodium.

By March 1986, the patient required 120 mg of furosemide daily to maintain proper fluid balance. He never complained of chest pain nor did he have any acute episodes of dyspnea. Unfortunately, his BP became poorly controlled again on furosemide, pindolol, and prazosin. In addition, he complained of fatigue and mild depressive symptoms. The prazosin was tapered over 3 days and captopril, 6.25 mg, was administered in the office 24 hr after his last dose of furosemide. The BP fell asymptomatically from

160/102 to 135/85 mm Hg in 1 hr. Captopril therapy was continued at 6.25 mg t.i.d. and the furosemide and potassium were reduced (40 mg b.i.d. and 20 mEq q.o.d., respectively). One week later the patient felt remarkably better—his BP was 140/88 mm Hg, heart rate was 80 bpm, and there were no physical signs of CHF. The serum sodium was 138 mEq/liter, potassium 5.0 mEq/liter, creatinine 1.9 mg/dl, and blood urea nitrogen 26 mg/dl. The potassium was discontinued and the furosemide was reduced again to 20 mg b.i.d. Over the course of the next 6 months, the captopril dose was increased to 12.5 mg t.i.d. and he remained clinically stable.

A. Comments

It is not unlikely to see an older patient with a long history of hypertension develop CHF. Hypertension remains a leading risk factor for the development of CHF, especially in individuals with left ventricular hypertrophy. Mild-to-moderate renal impairment is also relatively common in CHF and may be related to poor forward flow from the heart and decreased renal blood flow. However, the diagnosis of renovascular disease should always be considered in an elderly hypertensive patient with depressed renal function.

The patient in this case report had both abnormal systolic and diastolic function as assessed by radionuclide ventriculography. As mentioned in Chapter 1, approximately 30–40% of hypertensive patients with CHF have perfectly normal systolic function. Thus, in these individuals it is abnormal *diastolic* function that contributes to their left ventricular dysfunction. Digitalis preparations are unlikely to improve the symptoms in these patients at all. Furthermore, patients with diastolic dysfunction may not respond that well to increased diuretics or drugs that strictly induce afterload reduction. In order to improve diastolic filling time, beta-adrenergic blocking agents or calcium channel blockers are most beneficial. However, the beta-blockers should not be started without first obtaining data on ventricular function.

In the presence of systolic dysfunction, the diuretics, digitalis preparations, angiotensin-converting enzyme (ACE) inhibitors, and other vasodilators are all potentially helpful, alone or in combination. If coronary artery disease coexists with the CHF, nitrates and calcium channel blockers are also of potential benefit since myocardial ischemia may induce left ventricular dysfunction. The use of the various pharmacological agents for hypertensive patients with CHF is discussed in detail in subsequent sections of this chapter.

II. HEMODYNAMIC CONSIDERATIONS IN PATIENTS WITH HEART FAILURE

A variety of hemodynamic abnormalities are present in CHF (Table 6.1), which may be mostly compensatory in nature rather than causative. Left ventricular hypertrophy (LVH) nearly always precedes symptomatic CHF, and in hypertensive patients the increased wall thickness is seen for several years prior to any dilation of the ventricle. Thus, one might say that in hypertensive patients, LVH is the result of chronic pressure overload. The hypertrophy leads to premature myocardial ischemia and dysfunction that is strongly associated with the development of CHF. In nonhypertensive patients with CHF, hypertrophy is generally thought to be a compensatory mechanism in CHF.

With chronic heart failure, there is renal retention of salt and water that leads to expansion of the plasma volume and subse-

Table 6.1 Hemodynamic Adaptation in Congestive Heart Failure

Ventricular hypertrophy
Elevation of ventricular filling pressure
Activation of the renin-angiotensin system
Increased sympathetic nervous system activity
Redistribution of blood flow (to maintain flow to brain and heart)
Increased atrial naturietic factor (however, responsiveness is impaired in patients with CHF)

---

quently to an elevation of cardiac output (Starling's principle). As the intravascular volume increases, the ventricle is no longer capable of maintaining the cardiac output, and pulmonary vascular congestion develops. In recent years, it has been recognized that patients with chronic CHF have increased plasma renin activity, increased atrial naturietic factor production, and decreased plasma sodium levels. The serum sodium level has become recognized as an important prognostic factor in patients with CHF. In a study of 203 CHF patients reported by Lee and Packer from New York, individuals with serum sodium concentrations under 137 mEq/liter had a median survival time of approximately half of the time observed in patients with normal sodium concentrations. As will be discussed later, this finding may have implications for certain drug therapies.

Another neuroendocrine abnormality recognized to have prognostic significance in patients with CHF is elevated levels of norepinephrine in the plasma. The level of the plasma norepinephrine levels correlates with the severity of the CHF. However, catecholamine levels in the plasma are not actually related to levels of myocardial catecholamines; thus the sensitivity and numbers of beta-receptors in the heart may be more important. For example, it is generally accepted that the number of beta-1 receptors and the sensitivity of the beta-1 receptors are reduced with age *and* in patients with CHF.

Another important hemodynamic adaptation in CHF is changes in regional vascular beds. Even though the cardiac output may be significantly reduced, blood flow to the heart and brain is generally maintained. On the other hand, blood flow to the kidneys, intestines, and periphery may be greatly reduced. Increased renal vascular resistance causes reduced blood flow to the nephron in severe CHF, leading to the sodium and water retention mentioned above. Another effect triggered when the renal perfusion pressure is reduced and sympathetic drive increases is production of the potent vasoconstrictor angiotensin II (via the renin-angiotensin axis).

III. MAJOR CAUSES OF CHF IN HYPERTENSIVE PATIENTS

The major cause of acute CHF in any patient is severe myocardial ischemia or myocardial infarction. Occasionally, through 24-hr BP monitoring, we have seen patients who develop marked increases of the BP just prior to acute symptoms of pulmonary vascular congestion. It is unclear whether these patients are actually developing a "stiff" ventricle from increased wall tension or whether ischemia is present concomitant with the accelerated BP. If the mechanism for the heart failure is ischemia or infarction, then therapy is aimed at reducing the injury with thrombolytic agents and/or percutaneous transluminal angioplasty. In the event that accelerated hypertension precedes the CHF symptoms, improved BP control will often result in diminished "attacks" of pulmonary edema.

There are a number of causes of chronic CHF and a discussion on this topic is outside the scope of this book. However, in hypertensive patients, ischemic heart disease and diastolic dysfunction are the most common causes of heart failure. Diastolic dysfunction has been best described previously in hypertrophic cardiomyopathy and hypertension. The importance of diastolic function in patients with dilated cardiomyopathies is not known. But in hypertensive patients with normal end-diastolic dimension, coronary artery disease, or in those with elevated heart rates, diastolic dysfunction may be the etiology of elevated venous pressure on both sides of the heart.

IV. CONSIDERATIONS FOR ANTIHYPERTENSIVE THERAPY IN PATIENTS WITH CONGESTIVE HEART FAILURE

The main therapeutic objectives in treating patients with congestive heart failure are shown in Table 6.2. Very recently, two major prospective studies have shown that the treatment of heart failure with vasodilator therapy prolongs life. The first study was a Veteran's Administration Cooperative Study (VHEFT) that used

Table 6.2 Major Objectives in Treating Patients with Congestive Heart Failure

Improve symptoms of volume overload (reduce/eliminate edema, prevent fluid reaccumulation)

Normalize hemodynamics (reduce BP and systemic vascular resistance, increase cardiac output)

Optimize salt balance (restrict salt in severe CHF patients, moderate intake in mild to moderate patients)

Reduce myocardial ischemia with drugs or surgery

Reduce mortality

isorbide dinitrate in combination with hydralazine as the therapy and the second study was using the ACE-inhibitor, enalapril in addition to diuretics and digoxin (the Cooperative North Scandinavian Enalapril Survival Study or CONSENSUS).

The main classes of drugs that improve CHF symptoms and lower BP concomitantly are the diuretics, ACE inhibitors, and vasodilators, such as hydralazine and prazosin. There are still few data on the effects of the calcium channel blockers in this type of patient or these types of patients and there are no reports on the effects of the calcium channel blockers on mortality in CHF patients as yet. New studies have been initiated with beta-blockers in specialized patient groups (those with dilated cardiomyopathy), but data are not sufficient to extent recommendations to hypertensive patients with CHF.

V. DIURETIC THERAPY IN HYPERTENSIVE PATIENTS WITH CHF

In patients with hypertension and CHF, diuretics remain an appropriate initial therapy. It is reasonable to start with a thiazide diuretic, since the diuresis with a thiazide is less brisk, and the duration of activity is longer than with a loop diuretic. Many clinicians favor potassium-sparing diuretics (Table 6.3) for avoidance of hypokalemia since potassium supplements are often not

Table 6.3 Diuretics in the Management of Hypertension and Congestive Heart Failure

Agent	Type	Typical dose[a]	Other comments
Amiloride	K-sparing	5-20 mg daily	Use only with thiazide
Bumetanide	Loop	5-40 mg daily	Brisk, short diuresis
Chlorthalidone	Thiazidelike	25-50 mg daily	Hypokalemia common
Chlorothiazide	Thiazide	500 mg daily	May need b.i.d. dosing
Hydrochlorothiazide	Thiazide	25-50 mg daily	May need b.i.d. dosing
Ethacrynic acid	Loop	50-300 mg daily	Rarely used, ototoxic
Furosemide	Loop	20-240 mg daily	Useful when renal dysfunction present
Indapamide	Thiazidelike	2.5-10 mg daily	Nondiuretic vasodilatory property?
Metolazone	Thiazidelike	2.5-10 mg daily	Severe hypokalemia
Spironolactone	Aldosterone antagonist	25-200 mg daily	Useful in liver failure
Triameterene	K-sparing	50-100 mg daily	May increase BUN; used in combination with a thiazide

[a]Doses typical for congestive heart failure and not just hypertension; always start with the lowest possible dose. In hypertension alone, diuretic doses should rarely be increased above the initial dose.

well tolerated and thus patients are not compliant. This is a particularly important issue if the patient is taking digoxin.

The thiazide diuretics in combination with either amiloride, spironolactone, or triamterene generally are well tolerated and effective unless the patient has significantly diminished renal function. In patients with significantly reduced renal function, hyperkalemia may be induced by these potassium-sparing diuretics. Spironolactone has been used alone in right-heart failure associated with the secondary hyperaldosteronism of liver failure. In this clinical situation, it does not have much effect on blood pressure. One of the unusual side effects seen with spironolactone is gynecomastia in men, either unilateral or bilateral. Triamterene, an indirect inhibitor of aldosterone, may cause a rise in blood urea nitrogen; this is not a serious problem, but may mask reductions in renal function. Another rare, but serious side effect of triamterene is the formation of renal calculi when the drug crystallizes in the distal tubules or collecting ducts.

The loop diuretics (bumetanide and furosemide) are not generally first-line drugs in the treatment of hypertension. However, in patients with diminished renal function or heart failure, they may be remarkably superior to thiazide diuretics for both removal of volume and control of systemic arterial pressure. Obviously, potassium supplementation must be used in combination with the loop diuretics since combinations with the potassium-sparing diuretics do not exist. Between 40 and 120 mEq of potassium is lost with average daily doses of a loop diuretic; thus frequent monitoring of serum potassium and adjustment of the oral supplementation is required.

In patients with intrinsic renal disease and congestive heart failure, sometimes a loop diuretic is not effective in maintaining a diuresis. At this point, it may be helpful to add metolazone, a potent thiazidelike diuretic, which works at a different part of the nephron and is additive to the loop diuretic. However, some of the most dramatic cases of hypokalemia that we have experienced have been on this particular combination of diuretics. Even with very low doses of metolazone, it is not unusual to see serum potassium fall by 30–40% in a few days. Thus, great care and monitoring is required as well as using the metolazone only *intermittently* in combination with the loop diuretic.

VI. ANGIOTENSIN-CONVERTING ENZYME (ACE) INHIBITORS

The renin-angiotensin-aldosterone system plays an important role in blood pressure regulation. Renin is a hemodynamically inactive enzyme which aids in the formation of angiotensin I (Fig. 6.1). Angiotensin-converting enzyme (ACE) cleaves two amino acids from angiotensin I to form angiotensin II, a powerful arterial constrictor. In addition, ACE is known to be *kininase II*, which is re-

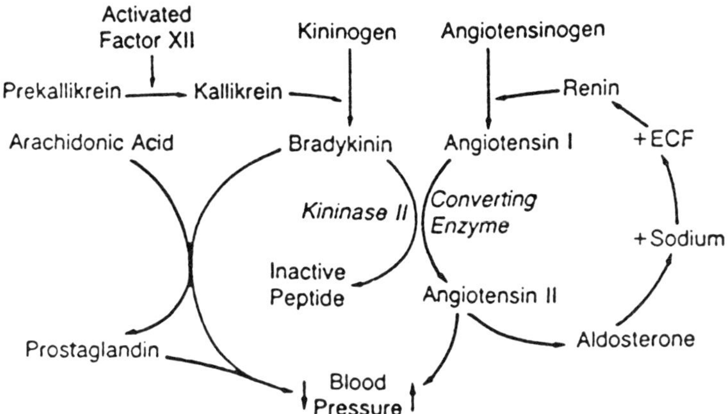

Figure 6.1   Relationship of renin-angiotensin system and bradykinin and prostaglandin systems to blood pressure regulation.

sponsible for converting bradykinin, a vasodilator, to inactive peptides. Aside from their weak vasodilatory properties, the kinins are associated with the direct stimulation of prostaglandin synthesis. Some of the prostaglandins are moderately potent systemic vasodilators. Thus, ACE inhibitors have a number of potential hemodynamic effects: By removal of angiotensin II there is reduced afterload and, by increasing the presence of kinins, increased engoenous vasodilator substances.

Not all of the ACE inhibitors are pharmacologically the same, however (Table 6.4). Some ACE inhibitors have a sulfhydryl group which attaches to the zinc ion of the converting enzyme (e.g., captopril) and others have a carboxyl group (e.g., enalapril). This may be important with respect to some of the side effects and to some of the potential advantages (such as removal of tissue-damaging oxygen radicals). Another important difference among the ACE inhibitors is the form of the drug. Some of the ACE inhibitors are prodrugs that require undergoing a metabolic alteration by the liver before taking the active form and others are in the active form at the time of ingestion.

Table 6.4   Pharmacological Differences in the ACE Inhibitors

Property	Captopril	Enalapril	Lisinopril
Zinc binding	Sulfhydryl (SH)	Carboxyl (COOH)	Carboxyl (COOH)
Prodrug	No	Yes	No
Maximal effect	1 hr	3–4 hr	7–8 hr
Duration[a]	4–8 hr	12–24 hr	20–24 hr
Oral absorption	75%	60%	30%
Usual dose, HTN	25–50 mg b.i.d.	5–20 mg daily	5–20 mg daily
Usual dose, CHF	6.25–50 mg t.i.d.	2.5–20 mg b.i.d.	25–20 mg q.d.

[a]The duration of action may differ depending on severity of hypertension (longer-acting in mild hypertensives) and absorption may be influenced by presence of food at the time of ingestion.

The first ACE inhibitor discovered was captopril; thus, there is greater clinical experience with this drug in both hypertension and heart failure (about 10 years at the time of this writing). Enalapril has been used fairly extensively for the past 5 years as well, and a number of heart failure trials have been conducted with this drug, including the CONSENSUS trial. ACE inhibitors lower BP in hypertensive individuals by reducing systemic vascular resistance and have little or no effect on cardiac output. In patients with hypertension and CHF, however, when systemic vascular resistance is lowered, cardiac output is markedly improved (Fig. 6.2).

There is some evidence that short-acting ACE inhibitors may be hemodynamically more beneficial than long-acting ACE inhibitors for patients with CHF. This comment is based on a sophisticated study by Packer and colleagues which compared captopril and enalapril in severe CHF patients. Two similar groups of CHF patients on diuretics and digoxin were placed on captopril or enalapril and then studied with invasive hemodynamic protocols. Both groups of patients improved markedly (subjectively and objectively) but the patients on enalapril had more episodes of prolonged hypotension (Fig. 6.3), worsened renal function, and more hyperkalemia than the captopril patients. This does not mean that

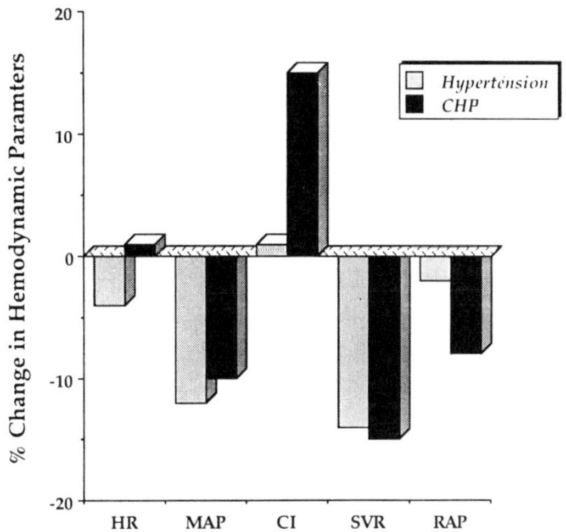

Figure 6.2   Differences in the effects of ACE inhibitors on hemodynamic parameters in hypertension versus congestive heart failure. The changes are approximate values and may differ modestly with the different agents. HR, Heart rate; MAP, mean arterial pressure; CI, cardiac index; SVR, systemic vascular resistance (index of afterload); RAP, right atrial pressure (index of preload).

enalapril is unsuitable for hypertensive patients with CHF. In contrast, the CONSENSUS study showed that enalapril significantly reduced mortality in heart failure patients and improved the quality of life.

It is reasonable to reduce diuretic dosing and potassium supplementation if possible prior to initiating an ACE inhibitor in CHF patients and to use the *lowest possible initial dose*. Diuretics stimulate the renin-angiotensin system; thus they induce a prime hemodynamic condition in which ACE inhibitors work. Special care in initial dosing of an ACE inhibitor should be given even to hypertensive patients without CHF who are currently treated with diuretics. In CHF outpatients, I strongly recommend giving the first dose in the office and letting the patient sit in the waiting

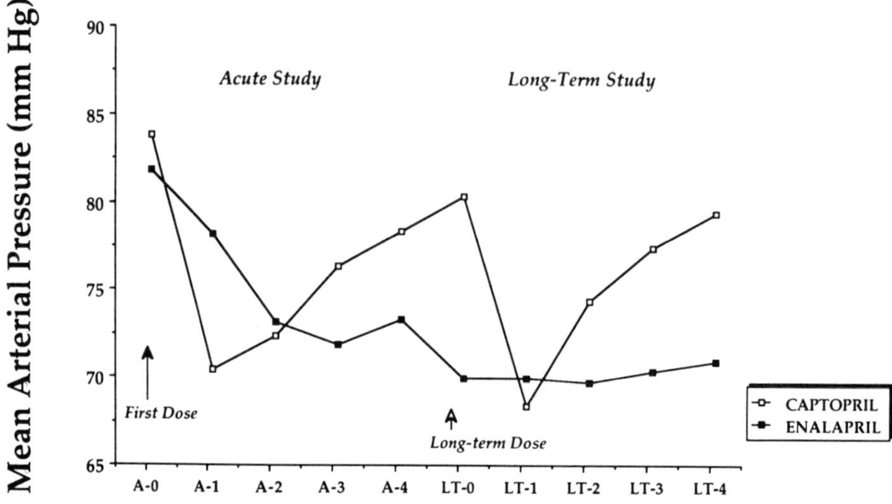

Hours After Drug Administration

Figure 6.3   Sequential changes in mean arterial pressure after a first dose of captopril and enalapril and after doses of each drug during long-term therapy in patients with chronic heart failure. (From Packer et al., *N Engl J Med* 1986; 315:847–853.

room; if captopril is used, the response will be observed within 1 hr. If enalapril is used, a few hours may be required.

A. Side Effects of ACE Inhibitors

When captopril was first introduced on the market, it may have received more "bad press" regarding side effects than any other new antihypertensive agent. During its development, it was studied almost exclusively in severe, resistant, and secondary forms of hypertension. Thus, patients with relatively complicated conditions received the drug and a number of adverse effects were reported, including proteinuria, leukopenia, and renal insufficiency.

However, over the past decade, as the use of the ACE inhibitors spread to all types of hypertension and to CHF patients as

Table 6.5 Nature of Side Effects of ACE Inhibitors in Essential HTN

Type of side effect	Approximate incidence (for all agents) (%)
Skin rash	2-6
Taste disturbance	1-3
Headache	2-6
Hypotension	2-3
Renal abnormalities	0.5-1.5
Neutropenia	0.04-0.06
Nonproductive cough	5-10

well, the incidence of side effects was found to be impressively lower than with most other antihypertensive agents. The side effects of the ACE inhibitors (Table 6.5) are relatively specific but differ greatly from those of other classes of antihypertensive drugs in that fatigue, sexual dysfunction, and depression are quite uncommon. In patients with hypertension and CHF, hypotension is more commonly observed than in patients with uncomplicated hypertension following administration of the ACE inhibitors.

VII. OTHER VASODILATORS WITH POTENTIAL USEFULNESS IN HYPERTENSIVE PATIENTS WITH CHF

A. Prazosin

This alpha-1 adrenergic inhibitor reduces afterload and, in patients with CHF, improves cardiac output. There have not been any long-term survival studies with prazosin in CHF patients as there have been with other vasodilators. There have been a number of reports that CHF patients develop tolerance to prazosin (tachyphylaxis). Now that other drugs are available for heart failure patients with hypertension, prazosin is less attractive as an antihypertensive agent that should be added to diuretics (and/or digoxin) for CHF. In severely hypertensive patients, prazosin (and the longer-acting alpha-1 adrenergic antagonists, terazosin and doxazosin) may be effective in combination with the ACE inhibitors. However, the combination of alpha-1 blockers and ACE inhibitors is quite potent, and great care must be taken to avoid severe postural hypotension, especially with the initial doses.

B. Hydralazine and Nitrates

While neither hydralazine nor a long-acting nitrate is that helpful alone, the combination of vasodilation and venodilation in patients with heart failure has proven effective and modestly reduces mortality in patients with severe chronic failure (left ventricular ejection fraction of less than 30%). In patients with ischemic heart disease, hypertension, and congestive heart failure, long-acting nitrates are likely to be used to relieve angina attacks. The addition of hydralazine in low doses may improve blood pressure in these patients, but care must be taken in its use since hydralazine will stimulate the sympathetic nervous system and may increase the heart rate. I would not favor the continuation of hydralazine as an antihypertensive or in a CHF regimen if reflex tachycardia occurred. This could be detrimental to this type of patient, and while reduction of peripheral resistance is sought after in both hypertension and CHF, a direct vasodilator in the absence of a beta-blocker may be arrhythmogenic.

VIII. FINAL COMMENTS

Congestive heart failure carries a relatively poor prognosis in hypertensive patients, especially if there is concomitant renal disease or the systolic function is severely impaired. The advent of ACE inhibitors has radically changed the management of heart failure with or without hypertension. Some studies suggest that some of the ACE inhibitors are superior to the digitalis glycosides in mild CHF patients; thus, it is likely that these drugs will become widely used alone or in combination with diuretics in the management of hypertension and all degrees of heart failure associated with systolic dysfunction.

REFERENCES

Cohn J N, Archibald D G, Ziesche S, et al. Effect of vasodilator therapy on mortality in chronic congestive heart failure. *N Engl J Med* 1986; 314: 1547–1552.

Consensus Trial Study Group. Effects of enalapril on mortality in severe congestive heart failure: Results of the Cooperative North Scandinavian Enalapril Survival Study. *N Engl J Med* 1987; 316:1429–1435.

Lee W H, Packer M. Prognostic importance of serum sodium concentration and its modification by converting-enzyme inhibition in patients with severe chronic heart failure. *Circulation* 1986; 73:257–267.

Mulrow C D, Mulrow J P, Linn W D, Aguilar C, Ramirez G. Relative efficacy of vasodilator therapy in chronic congestive heart failure: Implications of randomized trials. *JAMA* 1988; 259:3422–3426.

Omvik P, Lund-Johansen P. Combined captopril and hydrochlorothiazide therapy in severe hypertension: Long-term haemodynamic changes at rest and during exercise. *J Hypertension* 1984; 2:73–80.

Packer M, Lee W H, Yushak M, Medina N. Comparison of captopril and enalapril in patients with severe chronic heart failure. *N Engl J Med* 1986; 315:847–853.

Poole-Wilson P A. Current therapeutic principles in the acute management of severe congestive heart failure. *Am J Cardiol* 1988; 62:4C–8C.

White W B, Pandit R S. The antihypertensive agents: clinical pharmacology and therapeutic monitoring. *Clin Lab Med* 1987; 7:607–623.

7

The Hypertensive Patient with Disorders of Metabolism

Hypertension is one of the most common diseases managed by primary care physicians. Diabetes mellitus with and without renal dysfunction, hyperlipidemia, and thyroid disorders are also frequently encountered by clinicians in office practice. Since the aforementioned metabolic disorders are fairly prevalent, clinicians are often faced with evaluating and treating hypertension in these special patient groups. As is seen with hypertension, diabetes mellitus and hypercholesterolemia are associated with accelerated atherosclerosis; thus management of these individuals can be particularly challenging.

In this chapter, the focus is on management of hypertension when these disorders coexist in the same patient. Attention has been given to pathophysiology associated with the hypertensive diabetic, the hypercholesterolemic hypertensive, as well as the genesis of hypertension in hyperthyroidism. The pharmacological antihypertensive options in the various patient groups and how the drugs may affect the "other" condition are discussed.

I. HYPERTENSION IN THE DIABETIC PATIENT

A. Background Information and Pathophysiology

The close relationship between hypertension and diabetes mellitus has been recognized for over 50 years. The incidence of hypertension in Type I (insulin-dependent) diabetes ranges widely, but in individuals who develop nephropathy and renal insufficiency, the prevalence is 40–50%. In Type II (non-insulin-dependent) diabetes, studies have reported the incidence of hypertension to range from 10 to 80%. The marked variability in the frequency of hypertension in these different studies likely comes from lack of control of age, weight, and dietary habits. In any event, the incidence of hypertension in diabetic patients is higher than in nondiabetic individuals.

Diabetic hypertensive patients have been well studied for the past two decades to assess whether a common "link" between the development of hypertension and diabetes exists. Some of the pathophysiological findings that have been elucidated are shown in Table 7.1. When renal insufficiency associated with advanced diabetic glomerulopathy (seen more commonly in Type I diabetics) is excluded, the physiological disturbances in common between hypertension and glucose intolerance include obesity, abnormal sodium excretion, and insulin resistance.

The presence of insulin resistance in patients with hypertension has become a fascinating story that has been confirmed in a number of studies. Three conditions are now associated with in-

Table 7.1 Pathophysiological Findings in Hypertensive Diabetics

Insulin resistance (postprandial hyperinsulinemia)
Enhanced vascular reactivity
Increased sensitivity to sodium (abnormal excretion?)
Hyporeninemic hypoaldosteronism (hyperkalemia; more common in elderly individuals or those with nephropathy)
Normal plasma catecholamines

sulin resistance: Type II diabetes mellitus, obesity, and hypertension. Since two of these diseases often occur together, Ferrannini and colleagues from Pisa, Italy, studied moderate to severely hypertensive patients who were neither obese nor had glucose intolerance (normal 2-hr glucose response to 75 g oral glucose load). In their study, they found that nondiabetic hypertensives had marked impairment in the peripheral utilization of insulin compared to age-matched, healthy controls. Furthermore, the insulin resistance was directly correlated with the severity of the hypertension. One reason that this finding is of particular interest is that it is known that hyperinsulinemia may cause increased sodium reabsorption in the distal nephron. This may explain, in part, the sodium sensitivity of diabetic hypertensives. Other pathogenetic mechanisms associated with insulin resistance includes increased sympathothetic nervous system activity and abnormal cation transport (for example, increased calcium entry into the vascular smooth muscle cell accompanied by increased contractility (see Fig. 7.1).

In prognostic studies, the outcome of a diabetic with hypertension is substantially worse than that of a normotensive diabetic. Hypertensive diabetics with systolic blood pressure (BP) over 160 mm Hg suffer from an increase in most forms of macrovascular diseases, including congestive heart failure, intermittent claudication, limb loss from gangrene, transient ischemic attacks, and stroke. Hypertension does not seem to significantly increase the prevalence of coronary artery disease in diabetics, perhaps because the incidence is already so high.

Microangiopathy accelerates the decline in renal function seen in diabetic patients developing nephropathy. There have been a number of encouraging reports that effective blood pressure control (specific therapies are described later) in hypertensive, diabetic patients induces several favorable effects. Most significant is the long-term reduction in the rate of progression of renal failure. In one study of hypertensive diabetics by Parving and colleagues in Copenhagen, the rate of decline in glomerular filtration rate fell from 0.94 ml/min/month for the 2 years prior to the

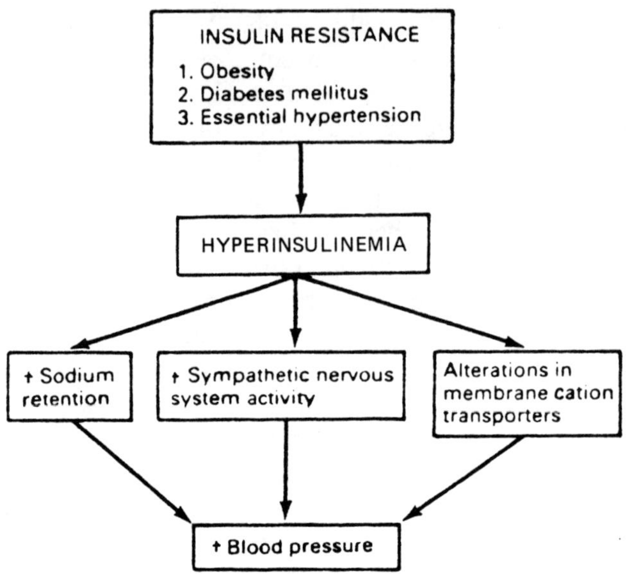

Figure 7.1   Mechanisms by which insulin resistance may contribute to an elevated blood pressure. (From Simonson DC, *Postgrad Med J* 1988; 64 (Suppl 3):39–43, with permission.)

initiation of therapy to just 0.10 ml/min/month after 4 years of effective antihypertensive drug therapy (Fig. 7.2).

Another favorable effect of antihypertensive therapy reported is reduction in proteinuria. As glomerular filtration rate deteroriates in diabetics, the rate of urinary albumin excretion rises progressively. In several studies to date, antihypertensive therapy has resulted in reduced albumin excretion in patients with diabetic nephropathy. It is of interest that in some studies there have been reductions in proteinuria unaccompanied by any changes in glomerular filtration rate. Finally, certain specific therapies (e.g., ACE inhibitors) appear to cause a reduction in microalbuminuria prior to overt nephropathy.

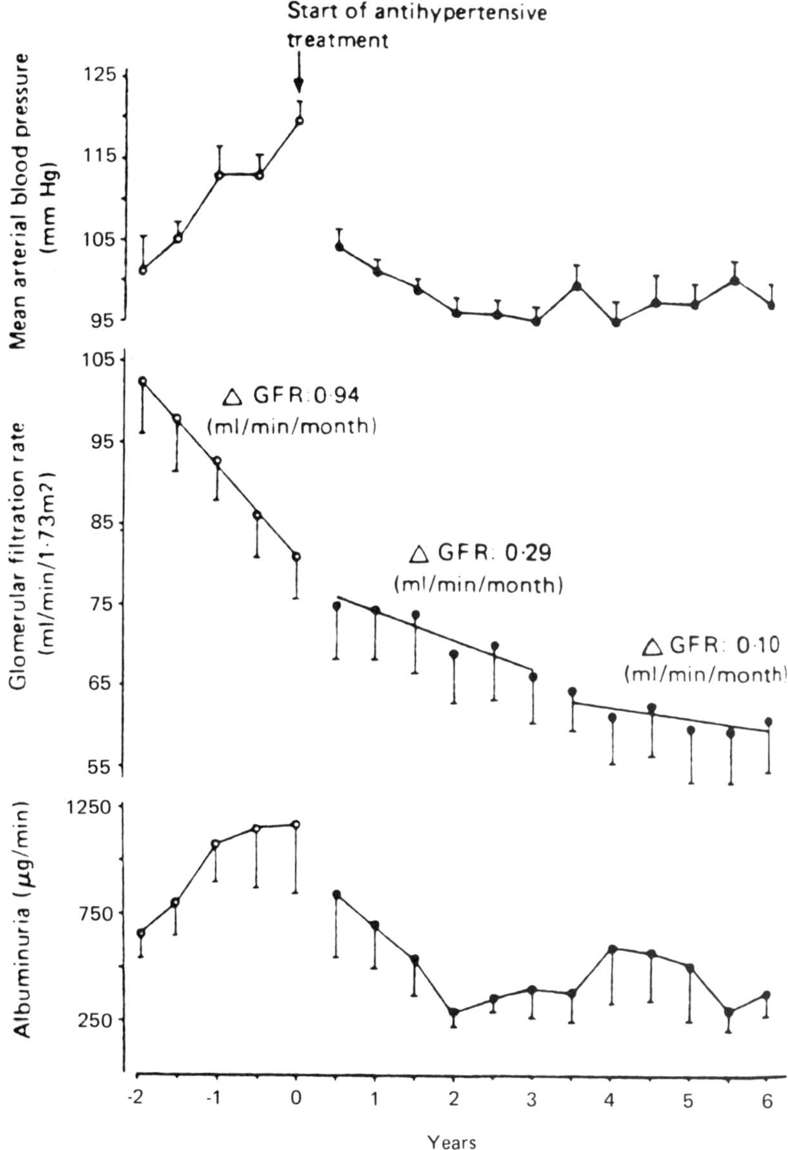

Figure 7.2 The course of blood pressure, glomerular filtration rate, and albumin excretion prior to (open circles) and during (filled circles) long-term effective antihypertensive therapy in Type I diabetics with nephropathy. (From Parving H et al., *Br Med J* 1987; 294:1443-1447, with permission.)

B. Therapy of Hypertension in Patients with Diabetes Mellitus

Nonpharmacological therapy can certainly be attempted in hypertensive patients with diabetes, and there are data demonstrating good BP responses to weight loss and restriction of sodium to about 2 g/day. However, one must bear in mind that excellent long-term BP control is essential in these patients. Reduction in weight is likely to improve both the BP and hyperglycemia, but quite often patients regain the weight, so they must be monitored regularly just as if they were taking antihypertensive drugs. If patients have a history of going up and down in weight and temporarily complying with sodium restriction, I would recommend using drug therapy for the greatest long-term benefits.

1. Diuretics

As shown in Table 7.1, diabetic hypertensives have impaired sodium excretion and are considered both volume- and salt-sensitive. Thus, diuretics may be quite effective in reducing BP in these individuals. Unfortunately, the diuretics are associated with a range of metabolic abnormalities that may have a negative impact on diabetics (Table 7.2). Diuretic-induced hypokalemia often re-

Table 7.2 Metabolic Disturbances Associated with the Diuretics

Hypokalemia—associated with impairment of insulin release (worsened glucose tolerance)
Hypomagnesemia
Hyponatremia—if severe can cause CNS symptoms
Hyperuricemia—often induces gout
Elevations in LDL cholesterol
Elevations in VLDL triglycerides
Hypercalcemia (uncommon)

CNS, central nervous system; LDL, low-density lipoprotein; VLDL, very-low-density lipoprotein.

sults in impairment in insulin release and thus aggravates glucose tolerance in Type II diabetics. Fairly often, we have observed Type II diabetics who have been maintaining plasma glucose levels under their renal threshold by dietary control but who lose this control once placed on diuretic therapy. Potassium-sparing diuretics should be used in diabetic hypertensive patients with normal renal function, but avoided in individuals with abnormal renal function who may have hyporeninemic hypoaldosteronism and high normal plasma potassium levels.

In the elderly, hyponatremia can be a serious consequence of the diuretics, inducing a variety of abnormalities of central nervous system function. Elderly diabetic hypertensives must be monitored careful since hyperosmolar coma (associated with marked hyperglycemia and dehydration) has been reported. While not a problem exclusively seen in diabetics, hyperuricemia is worth mentioning here since in clinical practice, it may be the most commonly observed "overt" adverse effect of diuretic therapy. Patients develop podagra (gout involving the first metatarsophalangeal joint) for the first time a few weeks after being placed on a diuretic, and there is not necessarily dramatic elevation of the serum uric acid levels (they may even be in the normal range for the laboratory). While they respond well to the usual therapy (colchicine or indomethacin), it is best to discontinue diuretics in patients if the problem occurs twice. The effects of diuretics on lipid profiles are discussed in greater detail in the next section.

As mentioned earlier, diabetic hypertensives develop premature macrovascular disease in the form of peripheral arterial disease, renal disease, and cardiomyopathy. In patients with renal insufficiency (serum creatinines over 2 mg/dl or 180 mmol/liter), the loop diuretics would be preferable to thiazide diuretics, and potassium-sparing diuretics are contraindicated. There are concerns that because diuretics increase blood viscosity, they should not be considered first-line antihypertensive agents in patients with peripheral vascular diseases, especially those with small-vessel involvement often associated with diabetes mellitus.

2. Beta-adrenergic Blocking Agents

The beta-adrenoreceptor blocking agents could be considered an initial therapy in a diabetic hypertensive; however, the concerns regarding a number of side effects may outweigh the benefits in the uncomplicated, mildly hypertensive patient. On the other hand, in diabetic hypertensives with coronary heart disease and normal left ventricular function, we often use beta-blockers as initial therapy. In these patients, we do attempt to keep the doses low, and as a general rule we avoid the nonselective agents. The cardioselective and intrinsic sympathomimetic activity (ISA)-containing beta-blockers at low and moderate doses are less likely to inhibit the adrenergic warning symptoms of hypoglycemia.

One relatively unrecognized side effect of beta-blockers is inhibition of beta-adrenergic-mediated insulin secretion. Thus, in Type II diabetics, the beta-blockers can impair insulin release and worsen glucose tolerance. In a controlled, randomized study by Dornhurst and colleagues, the beta-blocker propranolol was added to hydrochlorothiazide in a group of Type II diabetic men with mild hypertension, and several parameters of diabetic control were measured. As shown in Figure 7.3, both fasting serum glucose and hemoglobin A_{1c} increased significantly with the combination of the two drugs over the values observed with either drug alone. In patients with Type I diabetes mellitus, beta-blockers may have an effect opposite to that observed in Type II diabetics. Suppression of counterregulatory hormones (catecholamines, glucagon, etc.) by beta-blockers may accentuate insulin-induced hypoglycemia. As mentioned above, the nonselective agents may also mask some of the symptoms of hypoglycemia seen frequently in diabetics treated with insulin or oral hypoglycemic agents.

The presence of peripheral vascular disease in a diabetic hypertensive may also be a relative contraindication to the use of certain beta-blockers. The non-ISA-containing beta-blockers do increase systemic vascular resistance and may aggravate the symptoms of peripheral vascular disease, including intermittent claudication, cold, clammy extremities, and rest pain. ISA-containing beta-blockers such as pindolol and acebutolol and those with com-

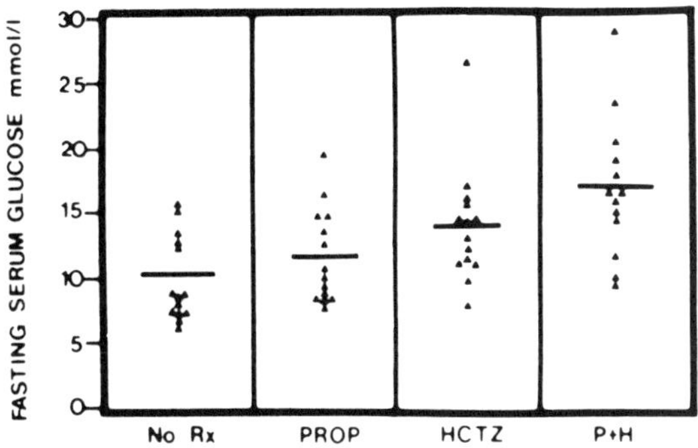

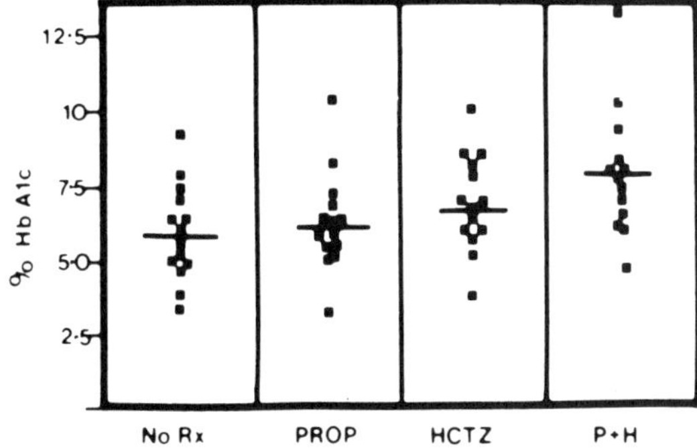

Figure 7.3   Fasting serum glucose (left) and hemoglobin A_{1c} levels at the end of four different treatment phases for hypertension in Type II diabetic men. PROP, Propranolol, 80 mg b.i.d.; HCTZ, hydrochlorothiazide, 50 mg b.i.d.; P+H, propranolol, 80 mg b.i.d., and hydrochlorothiazide, 50 mg b.i.d. (From Dornhurst A et al., *Lancet* 1985; 1:123-126, with permission.)

bined alpha-blocking properties such as labetalol are less likely to exacerbate diabetic vascular disease since they usually lower peripheral resistance.

3.   Alpha-2 Agonists and Alpha-1 Antagonists

The alpha-2 agonists (or centrally acting agents) include alpha-methyldopa, clonidine, guanabenz, and guanfacine. These drugs lower peripheral resistance and do not alter glucose homeostasis; thus many experts advise that they are safe and effective in hypertensive diabetics. Transdermal clonidine may be better tolerated than any of the other oral preparations since it has a somewhat lower incidence of dry mouth, sedation, and postural hypotension. Since methyldopa is relatively notorious for inducing sexual dysfunction in men, we have not considered it an appropriate first-choice agent in diabetics, a group with a high prevalence of sexual dysfunction.

Prazosin, terazosin, and doxazosin, are alpha-1 antagonists that also lower systemic vascular resistance, do not interfere with glucose metabolism, and have a low incidence of inducing sexual dysfunction. Thus, this class of antihypertensives has been advocated as an effective first-line therapy in diabetic hypertensives. However, since diabetic patients may be prone to postural hypotension from autonomic neuropathy, the alpha-1 antagonists should be used with some caution, especially the first dose. The first dose of any alpha-blocker should be as low as possible, taken at the end of the day, and the patient should remain supine for several hours after initial dosing.

4. Angiotensin-Converting Enzyme (ACE) Inhibitors

The ACE inhibitors (captopril, enalapril, lisinopril) have become quite popular as an initial therapy in diabetic hypertension, including in the presence of renal disease. There is increasing evidence that ACE inhibitors provide potential protection against glomerular hyperperfusion. Furthermore, the ACE inhibitors have been shown to improve glomerular filtration rate and decrease albuminuria in Type I diabetic patients with renal disease and Type II diabetics without overt renal disease. These beneficial renal effects, coupled with their very low side effect profile (especially with regard to sexual dysfunction and glucose tolerance), may make ACE inhibitors the class of choice in diabetic hypertensives.

In a recent study by Casado and co-workers, the ACE inhibitor captopril reduced excretion of albumin in diabetic patients

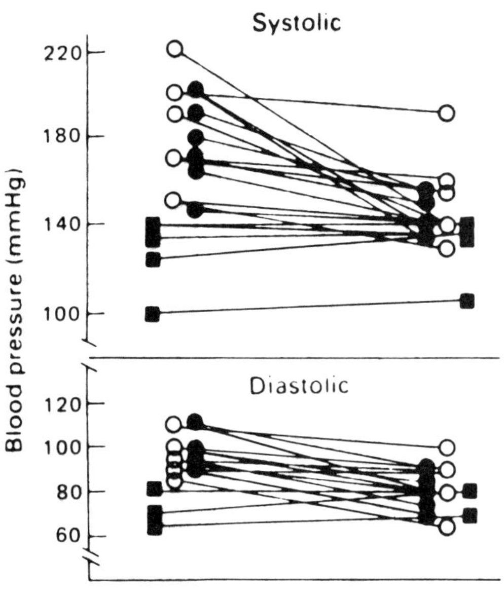

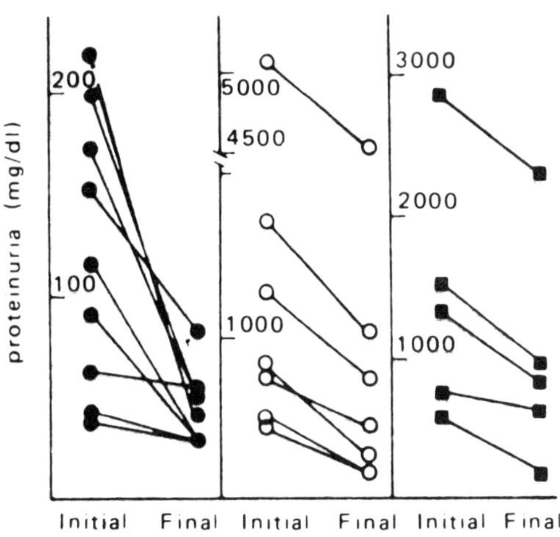

Figure 7.4   The effect of the ACE inhibitor captopril on blood pressure (top) and proteinuria (bottom) in three groups of diabetic patients. Closed circles, moderate hypertension and mild proteinuria; open circles, moderate hypertension and severe proteinuria; squares, normotension and severe proteinuria. (From Casado S et al., *Postgrad Med J* 1988; 64:85, with permission.)

with mild and severe proteinuria and in both normotensives and hypertensive individuals (Fig. 7.4). Thus, there appears to a direct renal effect of this class of drug independent of systemic arterial pressure.

The physiological effect of the ACE inhibitors is reduction in *efferent* arteriolar resistance that is regulated by angiotensin II. Thus, the ACE inhibitors reduce intraglomerular pressure by reducing the gradient across the glomerular space. This results in a reduction in protein excretion as well as delaying the decrease in glomerular filtration rate seen in diabetic hypertensives. Still caution must be exercised when using the ACE inhibitors in diabetics with renal disease, especially those with hyperkalemia, or concomitant renovascular disease. Clinically significant hyperkalemia is observed in these patients and blood chemistries should be monitored within 1 week of starting an ACE inhibitor in a diabetic hypertensive and renal insufficiency. We also discontinue potassium-sparing diuretics or potassium supplementation when initiating an ACE inhibitor in this patient population.

5. Calcium Channel Blockers

There are substantial data that demonstrate that calcium channel blockers (diltiazem, nicardipine, nifedipine, nitrendipine, and verapamil) do not impair glucose tolerance in hypertensive diabetics or in nondiabetic hypertension. Other advantages of the calcium channel blockers in the diabetic population include their lack of impairment of peripheral or central nervous system function and their potential improvement of peripheral blood flow in the extremities. The dihydropyridine calcium channel blockers are particularly potent peripheral vasodilators and therefore would be appropriate in patients with peripheral vascular disease.

Recently, preliminary reports suggest that calcium channel blockers have a glomerular effect opposite to that seen with the ACE inhibitors. The glomerular flow rate and renal blood flow may increase following use of calcium channel blockers and may be enhanced in patients with renal impairment. This may result in greater excretion of albumin in the urine. The long-term effects of calcium channel blockers on diabetic nephropathy are not fully known at present.

C. Summary of the Treatment of Hypertensive Diabetics

The main considerations for choosing an antihypertensive agent in a diabetic patient include efficacy and effects on glucose homeostasis, peripheral blood flow, and renal function. As discussed, diabetics may become particularly complicated if peripheral vascular, cardiac, or renal disease is present. Most of the antihypertensive drugs can be used as an initial therapy but certainly the potential side effects of some of them reduce their standing as a first choice (Table 7.3).

Table 7.3   Summary of Potential Benefits and Side Effects of the Antihypertensive Agents in Hypertensive Diabetics

Class of drug	Potential problems	Special benefits
Diuretics (thiazides)	Worsen glucose tolerance, sexual dysfunction	—
Alpha-2 agonists	Fatigue, sexual dysfunction, dry mouth	—
Alpha-1-blockers	Postural hypotension	Favorable lipid effects
ACE inhibitors	Hyperkalemia, worsen renal function	Beneficial renal effects
Beta-blockers	Worsen glucose tolerance with diuretics, mask hypoglycemia, aggrave peripheral vascular disease	Useful in CAD
Calcium channel blockers	Increase protein excretion	Peripheral vasodilation

CAD, coronary artery disease.

II. HYPERTENSION IN PATIENTS WITH HYPERLIPIDEMIA

Hypertension and hypercholesterolemia are both major risk factors that accelerate the development of coronary heart disease. Elevated blood pressure can cause local or generalized injury to the endothelial lining of blood vessels. The alteration of the integrity of the vessel wall predisposes it to excessive growth of intimal lining cells (so-called intimal hyperplasia) and aggregation of platelets. Hypercholesterolemia causes acceleration of the deposit of lipids in the areas of intimal hyperplasia and enhances atherosclerotic plaque formation. Thus, the presence of both hypertension and hypercholesterolemia dramatically increases the incidence of coronary heart disease, cerebrovascular disease, and occlusive disease of the peripheral arteries (including the aorta).

Some antihypertensive drug therapies have a negative impact on serum lipid profiles while others have either no effect or even modest lipid-lowering effects. Over the last decade concern has arisen from the lack of benefit of certain major classes of antihypertensive drugs on atherosclerotic vascular diseases. Thus, hypercholesterolemia may actually be so strong a risk factor for vascular disease that even the benefits of BP reduction may be negated if a drug increases lipids.

Five major lipoproteins have been identified that transport triglycerides and cholesterol and are associated with various

Table 7.4   Major Types of Lipoproteins in the Plasma

Chylomicrons—carry mainly exogenous triglycerides
Very-low-density lipoproteins (VLDL)—mainly triglycerides
Intermediate-density lipoproteins (IDL)—cholesterol and triglycerides
Low-density lipoproteins (LDL)—mainly cholesterol carried to tissue sites
High-density lipoproteins (HDL)—mainly cholesterol carried away from tissue sites

degrees of risk of development of coronary heart disease (Table 7.4). In general, the lipoprotein most strongly associated with heart disease is low-density lipoprotein (LDL) cholesterol. Since most hospital and commercial laboratories do not measure the LDL cholesterol directly, it can be derived from the following simple formula:

$$\text{LDL cholesterol} = \text{total cholesterol} - \text{HDL cholesterol} - \text{triglycerides}/5$$

The triglyceride determinations should be performed after an overnight fast, but fasting is not necessary for the cholesterol studies.

Depending on the expert group, there are slightly different classifications of hyperlipidemia. However, both the Americans and Europeans have had consensus meetings in the past 2 or 3 years to revise the recommendations for the diagnosis of hypercholesterolemia (Table 7.5). On both sides of the Atlantic, there has been agreement that in adults, cholesterol levels > 200 mg/dl (5.2 mmol/liter) require medical attention. This is based on data demonstrating increased coronary and thrombotic stroke risk in nearly all age groups when the total serum cholesterol is greater than 200 mg/dl. However, the total cholesterol value that has become established in the United States as the level at which intervention must be seriously considered is 240 mg/dl.

Table 7.5   Guidelines for Classification and Treatment of Hyperlipidemia

Total cholesterol	Triglycerides	Management
<200 mg/dl	<200 mg/dl	Recheck in 5 years
200-240 mg/dl	<200 mg/dl	Dietary counseling, weight loss
<200 mg/dl	200-500 mg/dl	Secondary causes?[a] Reduce carbohydrates
240-300 mg/dl	>200 mg/dl	Diet first, drug therapy if no response to diet in 2-3 months
>300 mg/dl	>500 mg/dl	Drug therapy

[a] Secondary causes include diabetes mellitus, alcoholism, estrogens, and some antihypertensive drugs.

The total cholesterol, low-density lipoprotein (LDL) cholesterol, and high-density lipoprotein (HDL) cholesterol each are individual risk factors for the development of coronary heart disease. Elevated LDL cholesterol and reduced HDL cholesterol are strong correlates of the development of coronary heart disease. Thus, levels of the LDL cholesterol *over* 130 mg/dl and HDL cholesterol *under* 35 mg/dl are associated with an increasing prevalence of coronary heart disease. The LDL cholesterol may be thought of as the lipoprotein fraction that carries cholesterol to tissue for utilization and deposit and HDL cholesterol as the lipoprotein that transports cholesterol away from tissue back to the liver for degradation, removal, or reutilization.

A. Mechanisms of Lipid Alterations by Antihypertensive Drugs

A number of mechanisms by which antihypertensive drugs alter lipid profiles have been postulated. Elevated blood pressure and serum lipids may be genetically related and the sympathetic nervous system may be a common denominator. *Lipoprotein lipase* is an important enzyme that degrades triglycerides to free fatty acids and aids in the production of the HDL cholesterol. In recent years, data have emerged that demonstrate that lipoprotein lipase activity is controlled in part by the adrenergic nervous system. Beta-agonist activity stimulates the enzyme's activity while alpha-agonist activity reduces it. Thus, beta-blockers may reduce lipoprotein lipase activity while alpha-blockers might increase the enzyme's activity.

Another mechanism by which antihypertensive drugs can influence lipid levels is through insulin and its counterregulatory hormones. For example, when insulin resistance is induced by diuretics, not only is there hyperglycemia, but also inhibition of lipid degradation, or lipolysis. This results in increased levels of triglycerides, LDL cholesterol, and free fatty acids.

B. Effects of Specific Antihypertensive Therapies on Serum Lipids

1. Antihypertensive Agents with Unfavorable Effects on Serum Lipids

The diuretics, beta-adrenergic blocking agents, and alpha-methyl-dopa have adverse effects on serum lipids. The thiazide diuretics hydrochlorothiazide and chlorthalidone increase both the VLDL and LDL levels in plasma by as much as 40–50% and 10–20%, respectively. Thus, both serum triglycerides and cholesterol rise with use of thiazide diuretic use. There are few data on non-thiazide-type diuretics but studies suggest that spironlactone (see Fig. 7.5) and indapamide have no deleterious effect on serum lipids. In most studies to date, HDL cholesterol levels have not been significantly altered by diuretic treatment.

The beta-adrenergic blocking drugs have heterogenous effects on plasma lipids, depending on their pharmacological properties. The nonselective beta-blockers increase plasma triglycerides by 20–40% and produce a fall in the HDL cholesterol by 10–30%. On the other hand, the beta-blockers that possess the property of ISA (or partial agonist activity) really do not increase the triglycerides much at all (0–5%) and may actually increase HDL cholesterol levels. The beta-1 selective agents are somewhere between the aforementioned groups of beta-blockers; i.e., they modestly increase triglycerides and modestly decrease HDL cholesterol. The heterogenous effects on the VLDL and HDL lipoproteins by the beta-blockers are explained in part by the different effects of the drugs on lipoprotein lipase. As stated earlier, if a drug stimulates lipoprotein lipase, such as a beta-agonist, VLDL levels will be reduced and HDL levels will increase. Thus, a beta-blocker with ISA, such as pindolol, will increase the activity of lipoprotein lipase, thus giving rise to more favorable effects on the serum lipids. In general, the beta-blockers have a neutral effect on total and LDL cholesterol.

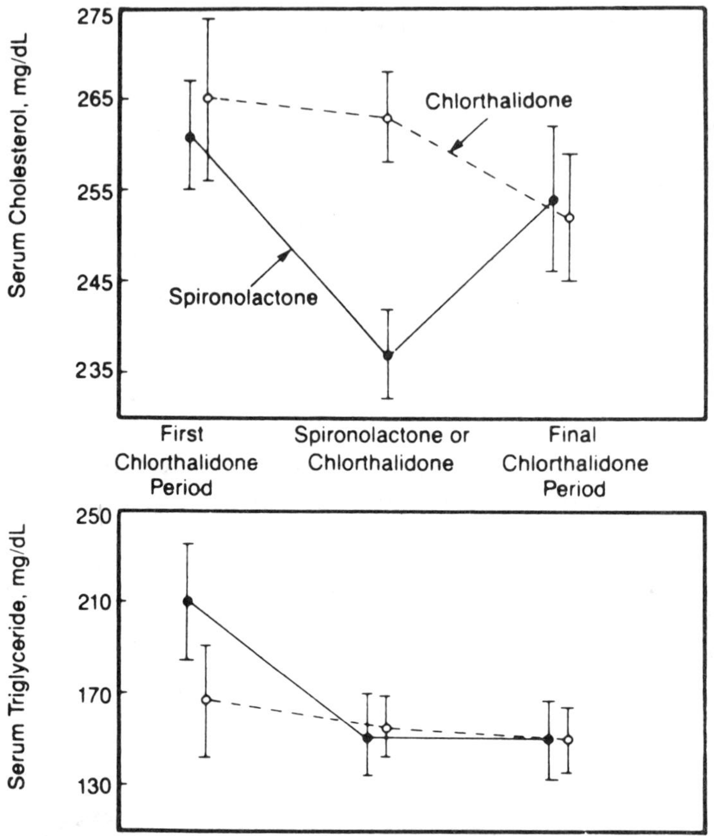

Figure 7.5 Serum cholesterol and triglycerides during each of three double-blind periods of diuretic treatment in 23 hypertensive men. In the second period, 11 men were switched from chlorthalidone to spionolactone and serum cholesterol levels fell significantly. (From Ames RP and Peacock PB, *Arch Intern Med* 1984; 144:710-714, with permission.)

2. Antihypertensive Agents with Favorable Effects on Serum Lipids

The alpha-1 antagonists prazosin and doxazosin and centrally acting drugs clonidine and guanabenz have all been reported to decrease total, LDL, and VLDL cholesterol without reducing HDL cholesterol. The major mechanisms that induce these changes are only now being worked out, but again there are data that indicate that alpha-adrenergic antagonists may increase receptor-mediated catabolism of LDL.

The effects of the calcium channel blockers, nifedipine, nitrendipine, diltiazem, and verapamil, and the ACE inhibitor captopril are more preliminary, but there are at least one or two reports for each agent suggesting reductions in total and HDL cholesterol. The calcium channel blockers have neutral or negative effects on the apolipoproteins, the molecules that form the outer coat of the lipid droplet and are considered markers for the development of atherosclerosis.

3. Antihypertensive Agents with Neutral Effects on Serum Lipids

The direct-acting vasodilators, hydralazine and minoxidil, have no significant effect on any of the lipoproteins in patients with hypertension. The ACE inhibitors, enalapril and lisinopril, to date have not been reported to have the same positive effects seen with captopril but this is more likely a function of timing of the studies than anything else.

There have been studies with combinations of antihypertensive drugs showing mixed effects. For example, if a diuretic and nonselective beta-blocker without ISA are combined, lipid levels are worse than on either drug alone. On the other hand, if the alpha-1 blocker prazosin is added to a thiazide diuretic, the net effect is no net change in total or LDL cholesterol. Thus, the alpha-1 blocker actually has a beneficial effect which negates the negative effect of the diuretics.

The summary of the effects of what is known about the effects of the major classes of antihypertensive agents is shown in

Table 7.6 Effects of the Antihypertensive Agents on Cholesterol and Major Lipoproteins

Class of drug	Total (%)	LDL (%)	VLDL (%)	HDL (%)
Thiazide diuretics	+5 to 10	+5 to 15	+15 to 20	−5
K-sparing diuretics	0	0	0	0
Beta blockers				
Nonselective	−2 to 0	−3 to 0	+20 to 30	−15
Beta-1 selective	0	−4 to 0	+10 to 15	−8
ISA-containing	−7 to 0	−8 to 1	0 to 4	+5
Alpha-1 blockers	−2 to −5	−5 to −15	−15 to 0	+4
Alpha-2 agonists[a]	−4 to −6	−10	−10	−3
ACE inhibitors	−5 to 0	0	0 to +5	0
Calcium channel blockers	−2 to 0	−8 to 0	−10 to +10	+5

[a]Data was for guanabenz and clonidine and exclude methyldopa. (Modified in part from Krone W and Nagele H, *Am Heart J* 1988;116:1729–1734, with permission.)

Table 7.6. These are generalizations based on a variety of studies with individual drugs within a given class. In some experts' opinions, there is not enough data on calcium channel blockers and ACE inhibitors to support their inclusion in the *favorable* effects categories. At worst, however, they have a neutral effect on lipid profiles similar to the findings previously presented on glucose homeostasis.

4. Fish Oils

In recent years, a good deal of interest has been generated in the effects of polyunsaturated fats on levels of both cholesterol and blood pressure, especially by patients. In my clinic population, it is not unusual for a patient to purchase large quantities of fish oil capsules, begin taking four to six daily, and then tell me about it 3 months later when he wants his serum lipids evaluated. I suppose most practicing clinicians have experienced this as well. The lay press should probably assume some of the responsibility for this since they are often eager to widely spread preliminary results of novel pharmacological trials.

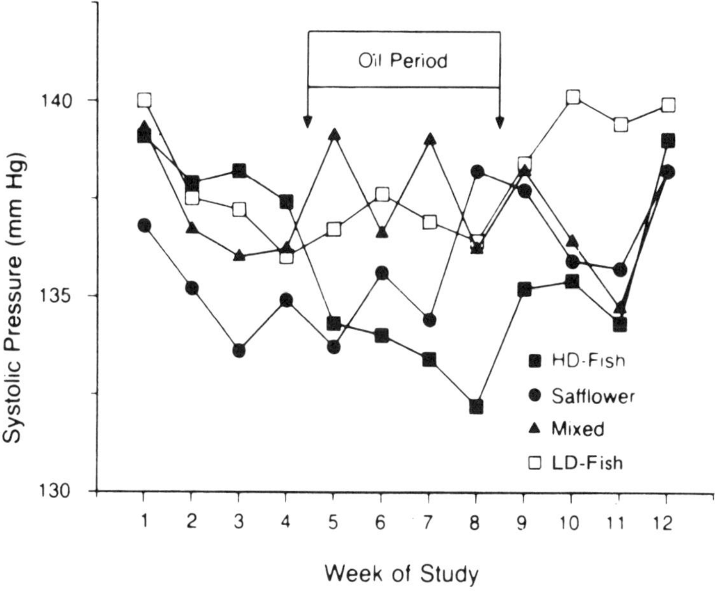

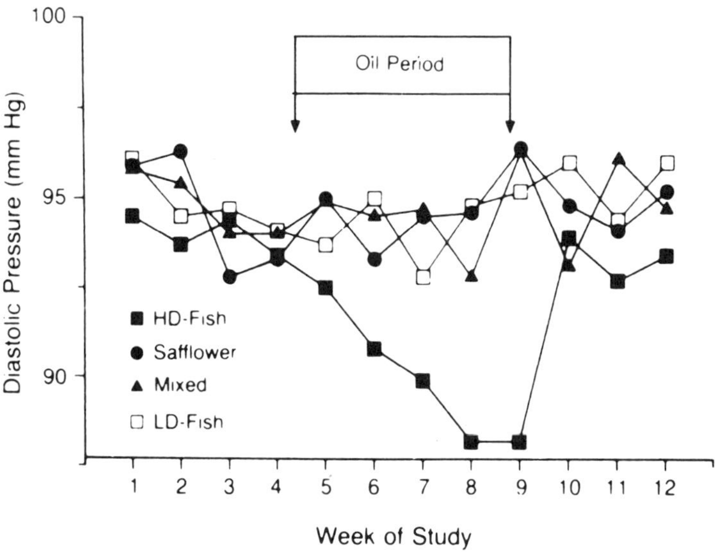

Figure 7.6 Changes in blood pressure on four different types of oils in 32 men with mild hypertension. The high-dose (HD) fish oil had a significant effect on systolic and diastolic BP, while low-dose (LD) fish oil, mixed (coconut, olive, safflower), and safflower oils had no effect. (From Knapp HR and FitzGerald GA, *N Engl J Med* 1989; 320:1037–1043, with permission.)

However, there has been one well-done, controlled study that demonstrated that the fish oils (which contain n-3 polyunsaturated fats) given in high doses (Fig. 7.6) lower BP; there are also data from other studies suggesting that marine oils also have beneficial lowering effects on LDL cholesterol and platelet aggregation. In any event, the amount of BP reduction seen following high doses of fish oils (50 ml/day) in the study by Knapp and Fitz-Gerald was modest and less than that observed with most antihypertensive drugs. Thus, whether this form of "nonpharmacological" therapy has long-term clinical utility in hypertension is not presently known.

5. The Effects of Antihypertensive Agents on Lipid Profiles

What happens in the serum of a patient is not necessarily a good predictor of the final outcome of that individual. For example, the beta-blockers with ISA seem to have a favorable effect on serum lipids and the beta-blockers lacking ISA appear to have a negative effect on serum lipids. In patients with coronary heart disease, though, it is the non-ISA beta-blockers that are cardioprotective and not the ISA-containing agents. It appears that control of heart rate associated with non-ISA beta-blockers outweighs the beneficial metabolic effects of the beta-blockers with ISA. In hypertension, the long-term significance of the negative metabolic effects of the diuretics and beta-blockers is not well established. In younger hypertensive patients with elevated total and LDL cholesterol levels, it seems reasonable to treat them with an antihypertensive agent that has a neutral or favorable effect on cholesterol. On the other hand, if the patient has a rapid resting heart rate, mitral valve prolapse, or anxiety, I would place the patient on a beta-blocking drug despite its potential negative effects on the serum lipids. I would use the same rationale in an older hypertensive patient with left ventricular hypertrophy or angina pectoris.

For certain patients, it may be problematic that some of the antihypertensive agents may increase LDL cholesterol or decrease HDL cholesterol. Thus, it is important to obtain fasting lipid profiles on all hypertensive patients, preferably prior to initiating anti-hypertensive therapy. If the patient has hyperlipidemia and no other concomitant illnesses, the first-choice agent for hypertension should be one that has a favorable effect on lipids. Obviously, if there is a supervening problem, such as a recent myocardial infarction, beta-blocking agents may be advisable, and that individual's serum lipids should be evaluated after a few months on therapy to assess whether an important change has occurred.

III. HYPERTENSION AND DISEASES OF THE THYROID

Elevated levels of the thyroid hormones may induce a marked increase in the systolic blood pressure. Triiodothyroidine (T_3) is believed to sensitize the myocardium to the catecholamines, thus producing increased myocardial contractility and increased cardiac index. When the circulating thyroxine (T_4) and T_3 are elevated because of Graves' disease, toxic adenoma, or the acute phase of thyroiditis, patients usually have a number of constitutional symptoms that suggest the diagnosis. However, not uncommonly it is an elevated BP, rather than weight loss, heat intolerance, palpitations, or tremor, that may be the first physical sign detected in a patient with hyperthyroidism.

In hyperthyroid patients, the systolic BP is usually elevated while the diastolic BP is normal or even low, so the pulse pressure is substantially increased. A typical BP would be 180–190/65–70 mm Hg accompanied by an elevated heart rate. The etiology of the hyperthyroidism has no major significance since any cause of hyperthyroxinemia (Table 7.7) can induce the hyperdynamic state.

The treatment of choice of the hemodynamic abnormalities associated with hyperthyroidism is with beta-adrenergic blockade. Beta-blockers reduce both heart rate and blood pressure and also have a beneficial effect on the tremulousness and anxiety associated with thyrotoxicosis. In patients with thyroiditis, the

Table 7.7   Common Causes of Hyperthyroidism
that May Be Associated with Elevated Blood
Pressure

Graves' hyperthyroidism
Multinodular goiter
Toxic adenoma
Subacute or Hashimoto's thyroiditis (acute phase)
Postpartum thyrotoxicosis

---

hyperthyroid state is transient, so antithyroid drugs such as pro-
pylthiouracil or methimazole are unnecessary. In patients with
Graves' disease, beta-blockade may be unnecessary after 3 or 4
weeks of antithyroid therapy. It is always wise to taper the agent
(non-ISA-containing beta-blockers should be used) over several
days after determining that the patient is chemically euthyroid.
When hyperthyroid patients will be treated with radioactive iodine
ablation, it may also be necessary to use antiadrenergic therapy
until a day or 2 following ablation since occasionally there is significant release of T_3 and T_4 following cell injury.

REFERENCES

Hypertension and Diabetes

Ames R P, Hill P. Improvement of glucose tolerance and lowering of glyco-
hemoglobin and serum lipid concentrations after discontinuation of
antihypertensive drug therapy. *Circulation* 1982; 5:899–904.
Casado S, Carrasco M A, Arrieta F J, Herrera J L. Effects of captopril in diabetic patients with different degrees of blood pressure and proteinuria.
Postgrad Med J 1988; 64 (Suppl 3):85.
Dornhurst A, Powell S H, Pensky J. Aggravation by propranolol of hypergly-
cemic effect of hydrochlorothiazide in Type II diabetics without alteration of insulin secretion. *Lancet* 1985; 1:123–126.
Ferrannini E, Buzzigoli G, Bonadonna R, et al. Insulin resistance in essential
hypertension. *N Engl J Med* 1987; 317:350–357.
Parving H H, Andersen A R, Smidt U M, Hommel E, Mathiesen E R, Svendsen

P A. Effect of antihypertensive therapy on kidney function in diabetic nephropathy. *Br Med J* 1987; 294:1443-1447.

Simonson D C. Insulin sensitivity and the effects of antihypertensive agents: Implications for the treatment of hypertension in the patient with diabetes mellitus. *Postgrad Med J* 1988; 64 (Suppl 3):39-47.

Taguma Y, Kitamoto Y, Futaki G, et al. Effect of captopril on heavy proteinuria in azotemic diabetics. *N Engl J Med* 1985; 313:1617-1620.

Hypertension and Hyperlipidemia

Ames R P, Peacock P B. Serum cholesterol during treatment of hypertension with diuretic drugs. *Arch Inter Med* 1984; 144:710-714.

Ferrera L A, Maratto T, Rubbar P, et al. Effects of alpha-adrenergic and beta-adrenergic receptor blockade on lipid metabolism. *Am J Med* 1986; 80 (Suppl 2A):104-108.

Knapp H R, FitzGerald G A. The antihypertensive effects of fish oil: A controlled study of polyunsaturated fatty acid supplements in essential hypertension. *N Engl J Med* 1989; 320:1037-1043.

Krone W, Nagele H. Effects of antihypertensives on plasma lipids and lipoprotein metabolism. *Am Heart J* 1988; 116:1729-1734.

Ross R. The pathogenesis of atherosclerosis—An update. *N Engl J Med* 1986; 314:488-500.

Hypertension and Thyroid Disorders

Amidi M, Leon D F, DeGroot W J, Kroetz F W, Leonard J J. Effect of the thyroid state on myocardial contractility and ventricular ejection rate in man. *Circulation* 1968; 38:229-239.

Fowler N O. High-cardiac output states. In: *The Heart* (Hurst J W, ed), McGraw-Hill, New York, pp. 477-488.

White W B, Andreoli J W. Painless post-partum thyroiditis seen initially as severe hypertension. *Am J Obstetr Gynecol* 1984; 148:346-347.

8

Management of Hypertension in Patients with Pulmonary Diseases

One important reason for inclusion of a chapter on pulmonary disorders and hypertension is that certain lung diseases, including emphysema, chronic bronchitis, and bronchial asthma, may have an important influence on the management of hypertension. As mentioned earlier (Chapter 1), cigarette smoking not only worsens the prognosis in hypertension, but may also influence the effects of certain antihypertensive treatments—thus, this topic is reviewed briefly in this chapter as well. Finally, a substantial amount of new information published in recent years has revealed important epidemiological and hemodynamic relationships between sleep apnea syndrome and hypertension. The impact of the relatively common problem of snoring secondary to obstructive sleep apnea on the pulmonary and peripheral circulation is discussed.

The following is a relatively typical presentation of a patient whose management of hypertension became complicated by his chronic airway disease.

I. ILLUSTRATIVE CASE

A 57-year-old man with moderate-to-severe essential hypertension and a history of intermittent bronchitis presented to a new physician in Waterbury, Connecticut. From the age of 17, he had smoked two packs of cigarettes per day but following the advice of his previous physician in Vermont, he had quit smoking 2 years ago. Frequently, when he developed an upper respiratory tract infection or if the weather became particularly humid with poor air quality for a long period of time, he would develop a productive cough and occasionally wheeze. Once or twice per year for the past decade he had required antibiotics for acute bronchitis, especially during the winter influenza and cold season. However, the patient did not consider himself as having chronic lung disease, so he failed to mention his bronchitic history to the new family practitioner.

On presentation he was taking hydrochlorothiazide, 25 mg daily, prazosin, 5 mg twice daily, and clonidine, 0.3 mg twice daily. He became fatigued for a few hours in the afternoons but did not complain of any other side effects typical for these antihypertensive drugs. On physical examination, the heart rate was 76 bpm, and seated, resting blood pressure (BP) was 160/102 mm Hg, averaged over three readings. Examination of the heart and lungs was normal. Pulses in the feet were diminished but palpable. Otherwise, the physical examination was normal. On laboratory examination, the serum creatinine was modestly elevated at 1.8 mg/dl and the electrolytes and blood urea nitrogen were normal. Chest X-ray showed no lesions, but there was suggestion of some chronic scarring at the bases of both lungs. Electrocardiogram showed increased voltage in the precordial leads and nonspecific T-wave changes in 1, aV1, V4–6.

Considering that the patient was fatigued on his present antihypertensive drug combination and that at a second visit the BP was 158/105 mm Hg, the physician decided that a change in medication was in order. He had also recently read that clonidine and prazosin were not that effective in combination since the centrally blocking properties of clonidine left little sympathetic activity for prazosin to work on peripherally. Thus, he decided to taper the clonidine (reduced by 0.1 mg b.i.d. every other day) and prazosin (reduced 1 mg b.i.d. per day) over a period of approximately 1 week, and to begin labetalol, an alpha-1, nonselective beta-blocker. The dose of labetalol was 200 mg twice daily while the hydrochlorothiazide was maintained.

On the second day following initiation of the labetalol, the patient began to notice dyspnea on exertion and intermittent coughing. Later that evening, he was wheezing and became short of breath at rest. He used an metaproterenol inhaler that he had had from the previous physician and stayed up, moderately short of breath, most of that night. In the morning, he saw the physician (he had called the doctor's service at 6 a.m. and was told not to take another dose of labetalol) and had scattered wheezes throughout both lung fields but was moving air well and not in distress. The BP was 170/110 mm Hg and heart rate 88 bpm. Cardiac examination demonstrated a 4th heart sound but was normal. An electrocardiogram was performed and showed no changes compared to the tracing taken 2 weeks earlier.

The patient was instructed to discontinue the labetalol and informed that this bronchospastic episode was most likely secondary to the new medication and that he should never take a beta-adrenergic blocking agent again. He was started on verapamil-SR, 240 mg daily, along with the hydrochlorothiazide. Two weeks later, the BP was 150/95 mm Hg and the heart rate 70 bpm. Dosing of verapamil-SR was increased to 360 mg daily, and after 1 month, the BP fell to 138/85 mm Hg. There were no further episodes of bronchospasm and the patient's BP remained well controlled.

A. Comment

In some patients without remarkable histories for bronchial asthma, but in whom there is a history of asthmatic bronchitis or seasonal allergic types of asthma, the beta-blockers *may* induce wheezing. As illustrated above, there were no physical findings or striking historical features to this patient that might be construed as strong contraindications to beta-blockers. Thus, any clinician could have first encountered the diagnosis of underlying airway disease in the manner shown in the above case.

Another important issue in the patient above regards the different pharmacological properties of the beta-blockers and their effects on the airways. Labetalol has multireceptor blocking properties, but the beta-blocking properties are nonselective and thus can induce beta-2 blocker-mediated bronchoconstriction. In patients with bronchial asthma, all beta-blockers, even those with partial agonist activity and beta-1 receptor selectivity, can aggravate the airway resistance and therefore are contraindicated. These issues will be discussed further.

II. SPECIFIC TREATMENT OF HYPERTENSIVE PATIENTS WITH CHRONIC OBSTRUCTIVE PULMONARY DISEASES

There is actually not a tremendous amount of up-to-date information on the pulmonary effects of the various classes of antihypertensive drugs. Some studies have focused on the effects of a drug or class of drug on ventilatory function in normotensive asthmatics while others have assessed both hemodynamic and pulmonary effects in hypertensive patients with chronic lung disease. Thus, the information reported herein is based on studies conducted in various types of patients on the angiotensin-converting enzyme (ACE) inhibitors, alpha-blockers, beta-blockers, and calcium channel blockers.

A. Alpha-blocking Agents

There have been two letter reports suggesting that the alpha-1 blocker prazosin may have beneficial bronchodilator effects in patients with allergic asthma. Recently, 17 patients with hypertension and either chronic bronchitis or bronchial asthma were systematically studied on prazosin monotherapy. The parameters of forced expiratory volume in 1 sec (FEV_1), forced vital capacity

(FVC), and forced expiratory flow between 25 and 75% of the FVC (FEF_{25-75}) were evaluated along with clinical records of wheezing, dyspnea, sputum production, and so forth. Following prazosin therapy, there were no significant changes in any of the ventilatory parameters; a few patients noted worsening of wheezing, but this study was not double-blind and there were no alterations in cough or sputum production. Thus, the majority of hypertensive patients on prazosin had no change in pulmonary function.

There are more limited data on the alpha-2 agonists, such as clonidine. In one study, clonidine was administered to eight mild atopic asthmatics whose FEV_1 was normal at rest. These patients were administered incremental doses of histamine by nebulizer to induce bronchoconstriction (a reduction in FEV_1 of 15%) following pretreatment with either placebo or clonidine (0.2 mg). There were no differences in baseline ventilatory function on the placebo versus clonidine regimens. However, clonidine modestly enhanced the bronchial response to histamine by causing a greater fall in FEV_1 at the highest dose used. However, the results of this study may not be used to generalize to the populations of hypertensive asthmatics or those with chronic lung diseases.

B. Angiotensin-Converting Enzyme Inhibitors

There have been a few studies with the ACE inhibitors captopril and enalapril in hypertensive patients with chronic lung diseases. Recently, some of these have attempted to assess a possible link between the increased levels of plasma bradykinin associated with ACE inhibition and exaggerated bronchoconstriction in patients with asthma.

In a double-blind, placebo-controlled, crossover study by Sala and colleagues, captopril was evaluated for its effects on bronchial reactivity by methacholine challenges in patients with bronchial asthma. When inhaled, methacholine induces bronchoconstriction, and the provocation dose (PD20) that causes a 20% reduction in expiratory flow was assessed on 4 weeks of placebo versus

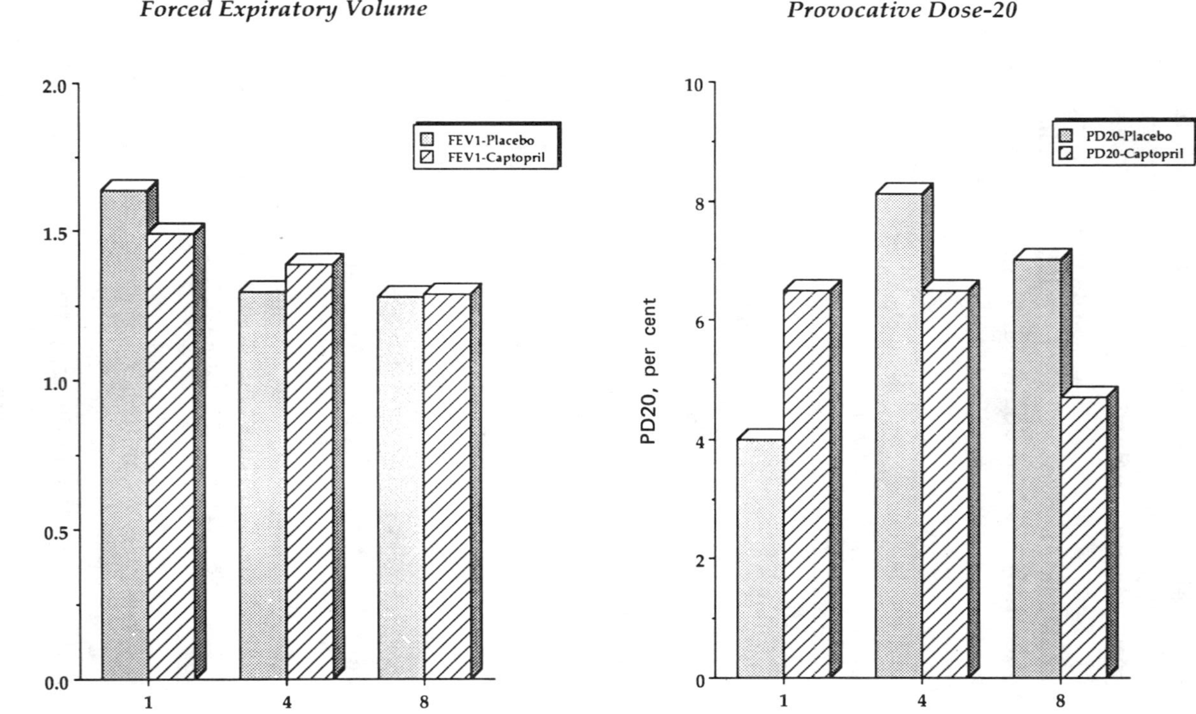

Figure 8.1 Effects of placebo and captopril on hypertension and bronchial reactivity (FEV_1 and PD20). None of the differences were significant. (Modified from Sala H, et al., *Postgrad Med J* 1986; 62:76-77, with permission.)

captopril therapy (Fig. 8.1). No changes in these parameters were observed. The authors suggested that hypertensive asthmatics could be treated safely with captopril.

In patients with severe chronic lung disease, pulmonary hypertension may develop in association with long-standing hypoxemia. Thus, it may be important if an antihypertensive agent reduces pulmonary vascular resistance as well as systemic vascular resistance. In an acute study performed in patients with chronic lung disease, hypoxemia, and pulmonary hypertension (pulmonary artery pressure > 20 mm Hg), captopril induced a reduction in pulmonary artery and wedge pressures as well as the systemic vascular resistance. A second group of patients with chronic lung disease had pulmonary function studies following 2 months of therapy with captopril and showed no clinically important changes in any parameter with the exception of a slight increase in vital capacity (10%).

Thus, it may be reasonable to conclude that the ACE inhibitors are relatively safe to use in hypertensive patients with asthma or chronic lung diseases. There is, however, an increasingly recognized syndrome of *ACE-inhibitor-induced cough*, which has been reported both anecodotally and from data obtained in clinical trials by authors in several countries. The cough seems to be a drug class effect and not drug-specific, since it has been observed with captopril, enalapril, and lisinopril, as well as some investigational ACE inhibitors. It has also been reported in both patients with hypertension and congestive heart failure.

ACE-inhibitor-induced cough may have an incidence as high as 10–15%. The cough is characteristically dry, may occur with greater intensity at the peak pharmacodynamic effect of the drug, and, surprisingingly, may not develop before the patient has been taking the agent for several months or even years! Before any major evaluation of chronic cough is performed, it is most reasonable to discontinue the ACE inhibitor, because in all cases that we have seen, the cough resolves shortly after discontinuation of the offending drug.

The mechanism of ACE inhibitor cough is not entirely clear, but some data suggest that certain individuals are predisposed to the syndrome, because they have hyperreactive bronchial airways 1 year after cessation of the ACE inhibitor. It is also likely that bradykinin, which is a smooth vascular muscle dilator, but also a bronchial smooth muscle constrictor, plays a role in inducing the bronchospasm. Inhibition of angiotensin-converting enzyme increases the circulating levels of bradykinin since its degradation is reduced. At this time, there is no evidence to suggest that hypertensive patients with chronic lung diseases are more likely to develop this coughing syndrome than hypertensive individuals with normal pulmonary function.

C. Beta-adrenergic Blocking Agents

The potentially serious effects that may occur if an asthmatic patient is administered a nonspecific beta-blocking drug were recognized soon after these agents came into clinical use. The nonspecific beta-blocking agents (propranolol, timolol, nadolol, pindolol) at any dose and the beta-1-selective agents (acebutolol, atenolol, metoprolol) at high doses can induce bronchospasm in patients with unspecified bronchospastic disease. The incidence of bronchospasm following propranolol is about 5–15% in patients with no prior history of obstructive lung disease.

The main mechanism responsible for the bronchoconstriction caused by these agents has been generally accepted as blockade of the beta-2 receptor in bronchial smooth muscle. Studies in both normal volunteers and patients with asthma have shown that metoprolol and atenolol can induce an increase in airway resistance. We have avoided using the cardioselective beta-blockers in patients with bronchial asthma, but have successfully used small, beta-1-selective doses of acebutolol, atenolol, and metoprolol in patients with chronic bronchitis and emphysema. The patients should be informed of the potential side effects of wheezing, coughing, or shortness of breath within a few days of initiating the drug and to seek medical advice if these side effects develop.

Newer beta-adrenergic blocking drugs, which contain selective beta-2 agonist activity (e.g., carvedilol and dilevalol, a steric isomer of labetalol), will soon be marketed in the United States and abroad. Chodosh and colleagues recently reported on the ventilatory effects of a single dose of dilevalol compared to equipotent doses of metoprolol and placebo in a group of normotensive asthmatics who had been treated with their usual bronchodilator regimen until 12 hr before the start of the study. The patients' FEV_1 and FVC were evaluated without intervention over 2 hr and following 2 hr during isoproterenol infusion (Table 8.1). The main findings were that dilevalol, with its specific beta-2 agonist activity, did not induce significantly more change in ventilatory function than placebo, while metoprolol significantly reduced FEV_1 and FVC compared to both placebo and dilevalol. The effects of isoprotenerol infusion on improving FEV_1 were moderately reduced by dilevalol, however. These data suggest that the beta-blockers with highly selective beta-2 agonist activity may be safer to use than cardioselective agents in hypertensive patients with stable bronchial asthma, chronic bronchitis, or emphysema.

Generally, since drugs like dilevalol or carvedilol are not available at the time of this writing, we have not been advocating beta-adrenergic blocking agents, including the "less" bronchospastic ones, as first-line therapy in hypertensive patients with chronic pulmonary diseases. In these patients who also have underlying coronary disease, angina pectoris, or recent myocardial infarction, we use the beta-blockers as first-line therapy with caution. The other clinical situation in which we might use beta-blockers

Table 8.1   Mean Change (%) in FEV_1 and FVC Following Single Doses of Dilevalol (400 mg), Metoprolol (200 mg), and Placebo in Asthmatic Patients

	Dilevalol		Metoprolol		Placebo	
	FEV	FVC	FEV	FVC	FEV	FVC
1 hr	−6	−7	−16[a]	−10[a]	−1	−1
2 hr	−5	−6	−16[a]	−12[a]	−1	−2
Peak	−10[b]	−10	−18[a]	−15[a]	−4	−5

[a] $p < 0.01$ versus the other groups.
[b] $p < 0.05$ versus other groups.
Source: Modified from Chodosh S et al., *J Cardiovasc Pharmacol* 1988; 11 (Suppl 2):S18–S24, with permission.)

in this patient group is if there is inadequate BP control on ACE inhibitors and calcium channel blockers.

D. Calcium Channel Blockers

As calcium channel blocking agents have been shown to have a general ability to prevent smooth muscle spasm in a variety of vascular beds and the myocardium, there has been considerable interest in their potential ability to prevent smooth muscle spasm in bronchi and bronchioles. A variety of calcium-dependent reactions affect various types of cells associated with bronchial asthma, including those in the smooth muscle and mucous glands, and mast cells and eosinophils. The mast cell appears to be affected dramatically by calcium-mediated reactions—there are electron microscopy data showing that following calcium entry into the cell, granules within the mast cell change formation and then release mediators through exocytosis outside of the cell. These mediators then result in bronchial smooth muscle contraction, move eosinophils to sites of inflammation, and aid in mucous gland hypersecretion.

Over the years, there have been data that suggest that some calcium antagonists, such as cromolyn sodium, when delivered directly to the airways block the mast cell mediators and thus reverse some of the bronchospasm typical of allergic or exercise-induced asthma. The calcium channel blockers used for antihypertensive agents (diltiazem, nicardipine, nifedipine, nitrendipine, and verapamil) are much less specific than cromolyn when given oral-

Table 8.2   Calcium-Mediated Reactions that May Be Involved in the Pathogenesis of Bronchospasm

Activation of mast cells—release of mediators in granules
Smooth muscle contraction in airways
Mobilization of eosinophils to sites of inflammation
Mucous gland hypersecretion—airway edema

ly and thus do not have such potent effects at the cellular level in the lungs.

One method of investigation that has been used to evaluate the effects of calcium channel blockers on airway resistance is in patients who develop asthmatic symptoms during exercise. The dihydropyridine calcium channel blockers (nifedipine, nicardipine, nitrendipine, and felodipine) have been fairly well studied in this regard. While results from studies are somewhat varied, most data suggest that these drugs offer a degree of *protection* in exercise-induced asthma. This effect may be dose-related, as shown in one recent study with the potent agent felodipine, in which a 10-mg dose of the drug caused complete inhibition of the exercise-induced fall in FEV_1 while 5 mg caused a lesser, nonsignificant effect.

Most studies have not shown any effect of the calcium antagonists on the resting bronchomotor tone. However, the calcium channel blockers nifedipine and verapamil have been reported in some studies to modify bronchoconstriction induced by histamine and other allergens. It is important to remember that the presently available calcium channel blockers have much more effect on the calcium channels of arteriolar smooth muscle than on those of the bronchi. The etiology of the reduced sensitivity in respiratory muscle is not known, but development of agents that selectively modify calcium transport in different muscle types will certainly be a wave of the future.

There have been few published reports of the long-term effects of the calcium channel blockers in hypertensive patients with chronic lung diseases. In one recent report from Bratal and colleagues in Sweden, cardiac function and blood pressure were assessed in patients with severe chronic lung disease following 3 months of calcium channel blocker therapy with felodipine. Their data demonstrated a fairly impressive (30–35%) improvement in cardiac output and ejection fraction (both right and left) in association with a dose-related reduction in pulmonary vascular resistance. In another study from Finland, eight hypertensive asthmatics were studied on captopril versus verapamil in a double-blind crossover fashion. Neither drug induced a change in the morning (before bronchodilator medications) peak expiratory flow after 4 weeks of therapy and BP effects were similar. There were also no subjective changes in asthmatic symptoms during the study period.

Thus, while there may not be particularly beneficial effects of the presently available calcium channel blockers in bronchial asthma, they seem to be safe for use as antihypertensive agents in these patients. In patients with chronic lung disease severe enough to induce pulmonary hypertension and depressed cardiac function, the calcium channel blockers of the dihydropyridine type may have potential benefit.

E. Other Antihypertensive Agents

The major reason that the other major classes of antihypertensive agents have not been commented on in patients with pulmonary disease is lack of controlled clinical trials. From clinical experi-

Table 8.3 Summary of the Antihypertensive Agents in Patients with Chronic Obstructive Pulmonary Disease

Class of drug	Pulmonary side effects/potential benefits
Alpha-1 blockers	None reported/anecodotal improvement of asthma
Alpha-2 agonists	Lack of data for both side effects and benefit
ACE inhibitors	Dry cough and bronchial hyperreactivity
Beta-blockers	Both nonselective and beta-1-selective agents induce bronchospasm
Calcium channel blockers	Potential benefit to patients with chronic lung disease and pulmonary hypertension and in individuals with exercise-induced asthma
Diuretics	Lack of data for both side effects and benefits

ence, diuretics do not induce any particular worsening of bronchospasm and are, of course, routinely used in patients with chronic lung disease and congestive heart failure. There also are no contraindications to the use of the alpha-2 agonists (clonidine, methyldopa, guanabenz) or long-acting alpha-1 antagonists (terazosin, doxazosin) in hypertensive patients with pulmonary disease.

III. ANTIHYPERTENSIVE DRUGS IN HYPERTENSIVE PATIENTS WHO SMOKE CIGARETTES

As mentioned in Chapter 1, hypertensive cigarette smokers are known to be at higher risk than nonsmokers for developing heart attack and stroke. Nevertheless, many hypertensive patients refuse to stop smoking and clinicians must manage them as best as they can. There are now a few reports that have evaluated some of the antihypertensive agents in smokers. In general, it is known that the beneficial effects on morbidity and mortality that have been attributed to the thiazide diuretics and the beta-blocker propranolol are largely negated by smoking. Furthermore, through a Veterans Affairs cooperative study, it was found that smokers had a lesser hypotensive response to the beta-blockers than nonsmokers. This study could not separate the possible effects of poor compliance from the actual effects of cigarette smoking, however.

The resting BP of smokers is the same as that of nonsmokers, but smoking is known to raise BP and heart rate acutely. This pressor response may occur even in patients who chronically smoke and the effect may last up to 30 min. Thus, a patient who has just smoked a cigarette in a waiting room (if you allow this!) or on his way to the physician's office may have a modest elevation (5–10 mm Hg) in BP.

A recent study by Mann and colleagues in New York evaluated the effect of beta-blockade with propranolol and alpha-blockade with prazosin on the pressor response to smoking. In this study, neither alpha- nor beta-blockade altered the pressor response to smoking, despite effective lowering of resting BP. They

Table 8.4   Considerations in the Management of Hypertensive Patients Who Smoke Cigarettes

---

Cigarette smoking may acutely raise BP

Prognoses for myocardial infarction, stroke, peripheral vascular disease, and renal artery stenosis are worse in smokers

Certain antihypertensive agents (e.g., beta-blockers) may be less effective in lowering BP in smokers

Initial therapy in hypertensive smokers should have positive effects on lipid profiles

---

hypothesized that in the presence of alpha-blockade, smoking caused a catecholamine-mediated increase in cardiac output, while in the presence of beta-blockade, smoking caused an increase in peripheral resistance.

In general, drugs that have a negative impact on lipids should probably not be considered for first-line therapy in smokers, since that could have a negative impact on yet another risk factor. The diuretics increase total and LDL cholesterol, and the beta-blockers can reduce HDL cholesterol; thus neither of these agents may be best suited for hypertensive smoking patients. The alpha-1 blockers, ACE inhibitors, and calcium channel blockers have either no effect or a hypolipidemic effect (see Chapter 7) and thus may be more appropriate for this patient population.

IV.   SLEEP APNEA SYNDROME AND HYPERTENSION

Sleep apnea syndrome is a heterogenous disorder associated with daytime somnolence, frequent periods of apnea during sleep (cessation of breathing for >10 sec), hypoxemia, and the development of pulmonary hypertension and cardiac dysfunction. Three types of this disease have been established: *obstructive*, usually secondary to a small hypopharynx and redundant uvula and posterior pharyngeal tissue; *central*, secondary to a central nervous system (CNS) disorder of respiration during sleep; and *mixed*, which is partly obstructive and partly a CNS problem.

Most often patients with sleep apnea syndrome are unrecognized by clinicians because the most common presenting symptom is excessive snoring. Since many individuals snore, patients fail to discuss it with their physicians. It is usually the spouse who notes the apneic episodes because he or she is kept awake by the loud snoring! Some epidemiologists feel that sleep apnea syndrome has been quite underrecognized and that it may be present in 5% of the general population (although it is more common in men than women).

There is an impressive association between sleep apnea syndrome and hypertension. In some studies of unselected hypertensives, the incidence of sleep apnea syndrome (defined in a sleep laboratory with concomitant electroencephalogram (EEG), electrocardiogram, oximetry units, and thermistors to detect air movement) has been as high as 15–20%. Conversely, the incidence of hypertension in patients with sleep apnea syndrome has been reported as high as 50%. When patient's have apneic episodes associated with significant hyoxemia, they have a surge in sympathetic activity accounting for a marked rise in BP. This occurs repeatedly during the night (in some patients, the sleep apnea index is 30–80 episodes per hour) and may cause a chronic rise in vascular resistance and even target organ damage.

We recently extensively assessed a patient with obstructive sleep apnea prior to and following corrective surgery. This patient had impressive rises in BP and systemic vascular resistance during sleep associated with apnea. Following surgery that corrected his redundant posterior pharyngeal tissue (uvulopalatopharyngoplasty), the apnea disappeared and his BP control and central hemodynamics (Fig. 8.2) were substantially improved. This patient, who manifested an extremely severe form of obstruction, went unrecognized as having sleep apnea syndrome for many years. Fortunately his respiratory and cardiovascular response to surgery was excellent.

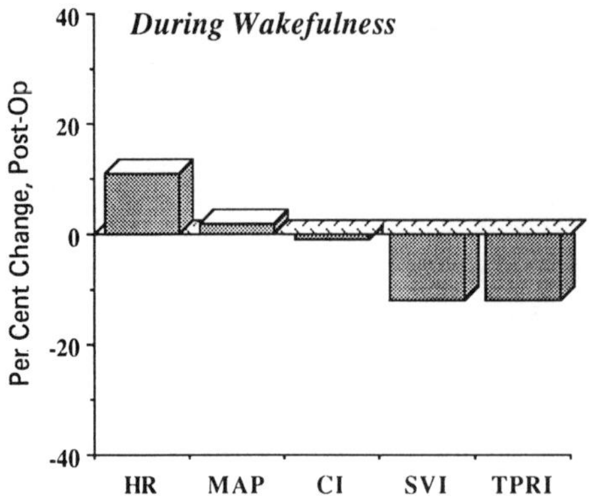

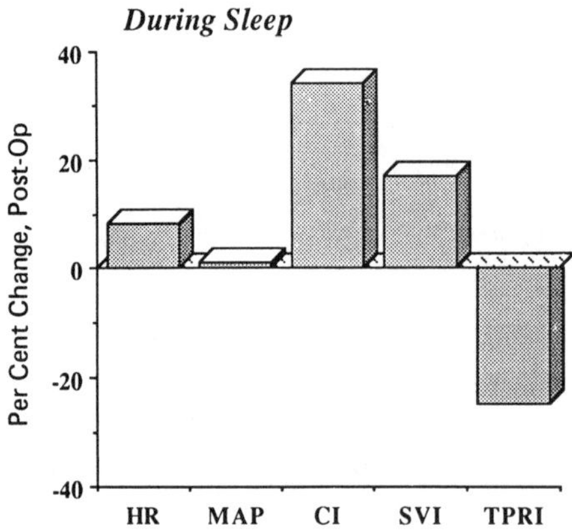

Figure 8.2 Hemodynamic changes in a patient with obstructive sleep apnea after corrective surgery. Note the impressive reduction in systemic vascular resistance during sleep (lower panel). HR, Heart rate; MAP, mean arterial pressure; CI, cardiac index; SVI, stroke volume index; TPRI, total peripheral resistance index. (From Lund-Johansen, P and White, WB, *Am J Med* 1990; in press, with permission.)

Table 8.5 Hemodynamic Abnormalities Associated with Obstructive Sleep Apnea Syndrome

---

Mild-to-moderate hypertension (epidemiologically linked)
Intermittent increase in systemic vascular resistance during sleep and apneic
  episodes
Intermittent increases in pulmonary vascular resistance during apneic episodes
? Left ventricular hypertrophy and early LV dysfunction

The sleep apnea syndromes may be associated with substantial cardiac morbidity, and recognition is important. The only way to be certain of the diagnosis is through a neurological and pulmonary workup in a sleep laboratory. In the near future, these studies will be performed on an outpatient basis since totally portable, ambulatory oximetry, EEGs, and air thermistors have been developed and are being actively researched at the present time.

REFERENCES

Bratal T, Hedenstierna G, Lundquist H, Nyquist O, Ripe E. Cardiac function and central hemodynamics in severe chronic obstructive lung diseases. Acute and long-term effects of felodipine. *Eur Respir J* 1988; 1:262-268.

Bucknall C E, Neilly J B, Carter R, Stevenson R D, Semple P F. Bronchial hyperreactivity in patients who cough after receiving angiotensin converting enzyme inhibitors. *Br Med J* 1988; 296:86-88.

Chodosh S, Tuck J, Basucci D J. The effects of dilevalol, metoprolol, and placebo on ventilatory function in asthmatics. *J Cardiovas Pharmacol* 1988; 11(Suppl 2):S18-S24).

Chodosh S, Tuck J, Pizzuto D. Prazosin in hypertensive patients with chronic bronchitis and asthma: A brief report. *Am J Med* 1989; 86(1B):91-93.

Lund-Johansen P, White W B. Central hemodynamics and 24-hour blood pressure in obstructive sleep apnea syndrome: Effects of corrective surgery. *Am J Med* 1990; in press.

Mann S J, Pickering T G, Alderman M H, Laragh J H. Assessment of the effects of alpha- and beta-blockade in hypertensive patients who smoke cigarettes. *Am J Med* 1989; 86(1B):79-81.

Patel K R, Peers E. Felodipine, a new calcium antagonist, modifies exercise induced asthma. *Am Rev Respir Dis* 1988; 138:54-57.

Sala H, Abad J, Juanmiquel L, et al. Captopril and bronchial reactivity. *Postgrad Med J* 1988; 62 (Suppl 1):76-77.

Tinkelman D G. Calcium channel blocking agents in the prophylaxis of asthma. *Am J Med* 1985; 78 (2B):35-38.

Xuan A T D, Regnard L, Matran R, et al. Effects of clonidine on bronchial responses to histamine in normal and asthmatic subjects. *Eur Respir J* 1988; 1:345-350.

9

Hypertension, Pregnancy, and the Postpartum Period

While obstetricians have always been the primary caretakers of common medical problems in pregnant women, it is reasonable for internists and family practitioners to have a good working level of information on high blood pressure (BP) in pregnancy and during lactation. On occasion, internists are consulted by obstetricians for advice on the proper administration of the antihypertensive medications. More commonly, a female hypertensive patient followed by a family practitioner or internist will seek advice on what to do about her antihypertensive drug(s) when she finds out that she is pregnant. Finally, obstetricians often turn over the care of most chronic medical diseases to generalists a few days into the postpartum period!

The following is a case of a hypertensive patient whom we followed throughout two pregnancies as well as in the postpartum period between the two pregnancies.

I. ILLUSTRATIVE CASE

A 26-year-old primiparous woman had had a history of mild-to-moderate essential hypertension since the age of 23 years. At the time of diagnosis, while she was living in Texas, a workup for secondary hypertension had been performed including 24-hr collections of urine creatinine clearance, catecholamines, metanephrines, and vanillylmandelic acid, and a renal scan. All studies were normal. Prior to the pregnancy, the patient's BP was well controlled on metoprolol, 50 mg b.i.d., and hydrochlorothiazide, 25 mg daily.

She realized that she was pregnant at approximately 6–7 weeks of gestation and presented to an obstetrician by week 8. Blood pressure at this time was 118/68 mm Hg. The hydrochlorothiazide was discontinued and metoprolol tapered over 3 days, and the patient was followed weekly for the next month. By the beginning of the second trimester, the BP had risen to 140/94 mm Hg and the patient was placed on alpha-methyldopa, 750 mg daily in three divided doses. This resulted in normalization of the BP (115/70 to 125/78 mm Hg) throughout the second trimester. At week 27 of gestation, the alpha-methyldopa was increased to 1500 mg daily because of moderate increases in BP both at home and during office visits. The patient continued daily BP checks with a home aneroid manometer and was instructed to report the development of elevated BP.

At 33 gestational weeks, the home BP rose abruptly to 180–200/110–120 mm Hg and the patient was admitted to the hospital for further evaluation. Initial physical examination revealed a heart rate of 80 beats/min (bpm) and a supine BP of 180/114 mm Hg. Abdominal and pelvic examination suggested a fetal size of approximately 1500 g and estimated gestational age of 29–31 weeks (confirmed by ultrasonography). There was +++ edema present in the distal lower extremities. The remainder of the physical and neurological examination was normal. Over the next hospital day, the patient did not improve despite addition of hydralazine to the antihypertensive regimen; the BP remained 175–190/105–115 mm Hg, and brisk tendon reflexes developed.

Urinalysis demonstrated ++ protein, the platelet count dropped from 243,000/mm³ to 128,000/mm³, and the serum transaminases were twice the normal values. A diagnosis of impending toxemia was made and the patient was delivered of a 1400-g female infant by Cesarean section. The patient was placed on a continuous intravenous infusion of magnesium sulfate and the methyldopa was continued. Fortunately, no large fluctuations in the BP or heart rate were noted during the operation and within 24 hr of delivery the BP was 140/90 mm Hg (Fig. 9.1).

Three weeks after delivery, the infant was discharged from the hospital and the mother began breast feeding (she had maintained milk flow with an electronic pump several times daily). The patient had decided that she wished to breast-feed her infant for several months. Thus, the alpha-methyldopa was continued at a reduced dose of 250 mg b.i.d. with fairly good BP control

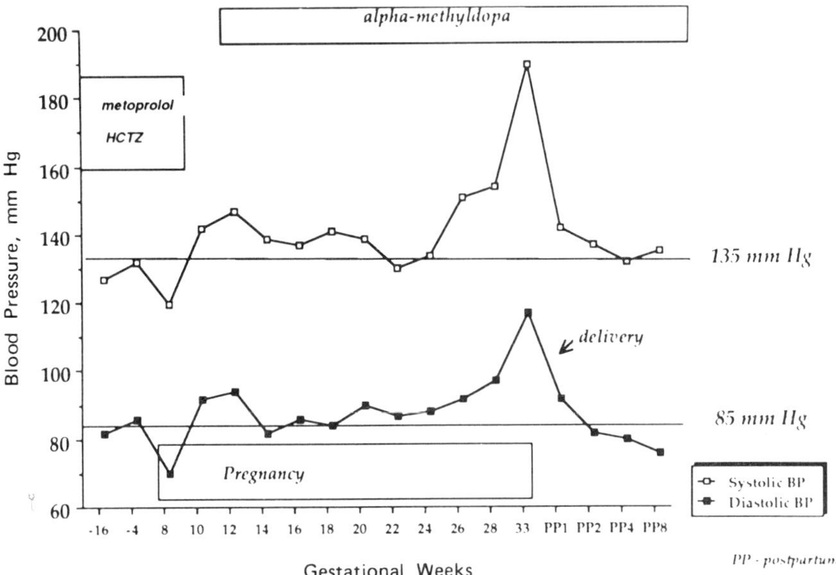

Figure 9.1 Clinical course and blood pressure levels in a patient with chronic hypertension during pregnancy.

(135/80–140/90 mm Hg). Levels of alpha-methyldopa in human breast milk vary but are generally in the order of 0.02% of the maternal dose; however, the relative dose to a newborn infant would be 20-fold greater considering the average weight of a newborn. No ill effects were seen in the infant over the next 6 months while nursing and there was totally normally growth and development.

The patient had side effects from the alpha-methyldopa of fatigue and lethargy, and after 6 months, the drug was discontinued and she was placed on atenolol, 50 mg daily. Over the next 4 years, BP control appeared quite good at regular office visits and through review of home BP measurements made by either the patient or her husband.

Last year, the patient again became pregnant, but at the onset of this pregnancy weighed 30 lb more than at her previous pregnancy. The atenolol was maintained at a dose of 50 mg daily and then early into the second trimester was increased to 100 mg daily when the office BP rose to 140/90 mm Hg. The BP came down to 125/80 mm Hg on the higher dose of atenolol, and the patient went to full term on the beta-blocker. A healthy male infant was born by Cesarean section with Apgar scores of 8 and 10. There were no problems in the periparum period with elevated BP. The first postpartum day, the atenolol was reduced to 50 mg and BP remained under good control.

II. CHANGES IN THE CARDIOVASCULAR SYSTEM DURING PREGNANCY

In order to treat hypertension during pregnancy it is important to be familiar with the major hemodynamic alterations that occur throughout the three trimesters (since this is the way that pregnancy is usually studied and reported in the literature). Normally, pregnancy induces a number of significant changes (Table 9.1) in central hemodynamics that increase cardiac function to keep up with the demands of the expanding uteroplacental vascular network.

Table 9.1   Hemodynamic Changes Occurring During Normal Pregnancy

Parameter	<20 weeks of gestation	>30 weeks of gestation
Blood pressure	Decreases[a]	Increases
Heart rate	Increases	Increases
Plasma volume	Increases markedly	Remains stable
Cardiac output	Increases markedly	Decreases
Stroke volume	Increases markedly	Decreases
Total peripheral resistance	Decreases	Remains stable

[a]Normal BP during pregnancy is <130/80 mm Hg.

An expansion of plasma volume occurs over the first two trimesters of pregnancy, accompanied by a 40–50% increase in cardiac output compared to the nonpregnant values. In women without cardiac disease, vascular resistance decreases in the first half of pregnancy, perhaps secondary to hormones and the erosion of maternal endometrial blood vessels by trophoblastic tissue. Reductions in both systolic and diastolic pressure occur at the end of the first trimester, remain stable during the second trimester, and then begin to rise again during the end of pregnancy (to prepartum values). Thus, for most of pregnancy, a BP of 140/90 mm Hg is not considered the normal cutoff. Actually, the average BP during the first trimester is about 105/55 mm Hg, so many obstetricians will begin to show concern with pressures over 130/80 mm Hg.

III. HYPERTENSION DURING PREGNANCY

Elevated BP during pregnancy falls into two main categories: pregnancy-induced hypertension (PIH) and chronic hypertension during pregnancy. The former term is used for the development of hypertension at any time during pregnancy (including around labor) in patients who were normotensive prior to pregnancy. Chronic hypertension during pregnancy means that the patient was hypertensive prior to being pregnant and continues to have elevated BP throughout the various trimesters. In chronically hypertensive patients whose BP elevates markedly during pregnancy (as shown in Fig. 9.1), the terminology most commonly used by obstetricians is that the patient has PIH superimposed on chronic hypertension. When seeing these patients in consultation, I have never been completely sure whether this is always correct since BP control may be lost for a number of reasons, including weight gain, volume retention, noncompliance with medications, and so forth.

Eclampsia or the development of toxemia of pregnancy suggests an entire syndrome, not just elevated BP. Findings in preeclamptic women include mild-to-moderate hypertension, hyperreflexia, albuminuria, abnormal liver enzymes, and occasionally hematological abnormalities, such as thrombocytopenia. If the baby is not delivered, eclampsia can develop and give rise to severe neurological complications, including major generalized seizures. The cause of toxemia of pregnancy is not known but morbidity and mortality from this disease is still alarmingly high. Obstetricians treat preeclampsia primarily with central nervous system depressants and delivery of the infant. A full discussion of the management of preeclampsia and eclampsia is beyond the scope of this book.

IV. ANTIHYPERTENSIVE THERAPY DURING PREGNANCY

Development and growth of the fetus is jeopardized in the presence of maternal hypertension, and several studies have now shown that good BP control during pregnancy lowers fetal risk. One must bear in mind that one is taking care of *two* patients rather than one when prescribing medications to a pregnant, hypertensive woman. Thus, good clinical studies of pregnancy hypertension have assessed both efficacy in lowering blood pressure and the ability to improve fetal outcome.

Therapy is usually tailored to maintain the BP below 130/80 mm Hg throughout the pregnancy. In a chronically hypertensive

Table 9.2   Nonpharmacological (Antihypertensive) Therapy of Pregnancy Hypertension

---

Prolonged bed rest (including hospitalization)
Spending >2 hr daily in the left lateral decubitus position
Sodium restriction (<2/day)
Mild sedatives

---

patient already on medication, the BP may fall during the first trimester secondary to the development of the uteroplacental vessels and the fall in vascular resistance. Therefore, usual doses of antihypertensive medications may require lowering. Later in the pregnancy, doses may require readjusting as BP normally increases.

Many obstetricians advocate a trial of nonpharmacological therapy before they will initiate an antihypertensive drug (Table 9.2). Often, they will even admit the patient to the hospital for a few days to assess the response to these maneuvers. At the same time possible distress to the fetus or signs of preeclampsia should be evaluated. Most common of these studies include ultrasound to assess development and a fetal stress test in which fetal heart rate is evaluated in different maternal positions.

Bed rest in the left lateral decubitus position is commonly suggested as a treatment for elevated BP and peripheral edema. The reasoning behind this maneuver is that the enlarged uterus often compresses the inferior vena cava, resulting in venous pooling distally and compartmental increases in intravascular volume. By spending a couple of hours in the left lateral decubitus position, the compression is relieved, allowing for normalization of the peripheral circulation.

The above therapies for hypertension may help in some patients. However, there are several problems with these forms of treatment of hypertension during pregnancy. First, they have not been systematically studied in a controlled fashion to assess efficacy and maternal and fetal outcome. Furthermore, not infrequently this type of treatment requires that the hypertensive woman cease all activities and stay in bed for several weeks or months. This is very difficult for many patients to do, especially if they are alone all day.

V. VARIOUS DRUG THERAPIES

The various antihypertensive drugs in pregnancy hypertension are summarized in Table 9.3

A. Alpha-2 Agonists

The alpha-2 agonists are among the best studied of all antihypertensive drugs during pregnancy. Methyldopa is an effective antihypertensive agent that has been widely used in treating all types of pregnancy hypertension. In England, there have been controlled clinical trials with this drug alone and in comparisons with other agents. More important, methyldopa is one of the few agents that have been evaluated for effects on perinatal mortality and morbidity as well as fetal outcome, in both the short and long term. In one large study by Redman and co-workers, there was an impressive reduction in perinatal fetal death (0.9% in the treated group versus 7.2% in the untreated group) in nearly 250 women with chronic hypertension during pregnancy. Maternal side effects of methyldopa were similar to those in the nonobstetric population and included dizziness, depression, and lethargy.

Several years later, 195 of the children born to the treated mothers in the above trial were evaluated by pediatricians for differences in a variety of physical and mental parameters. More than 7 years after birth, there was a small, clinically insignificant size difference between the boys in the untreated group and those whose mothers received methyldopa. There were no differences in other physical parameters, including sight, hearing, intelligence, or BP. Thus, this comprehensive long-term follow-up reinforces not only the efficacy of methyldopa in women with hypertension during pregnancy, but its safety as well.

Clonidine has also been evaluated in hypertensive pregnant patients in controlled studies. Blood pressure control is similar

Table 9.3 Specific Antihypertensive Drug Therapy in Hypertension During Pregnancy

Class of drug	Agents studied	Special features/concerns
ACE inhibitors	Only anecdotal reports	Animal studies show increased intrauterine death with captopril, fetal renal failure in humans
Alpha-2 agonist	Alpha-methyldopa clonidine	Reassuring long-term follow-up of offspring from mothers treated with methyldopa
Alpha-1 blocker	Prazosin (small number), labetalol	Neonatal depression, bradycardia
Beta-blockers	Atenolol, acebutolol, metoprolol, pindolol, propranolol	Neonatal bradycardia, respiratory depression may occur rarely
Calcium channel blockers	Nifedipine, nitrendipine	Limited data available
Diuretics	Thiazides, furosemide, spironolactone	Restrict use to high-volume states (e.g., CHF, renal failure)
Vasodilators	Hydralazine	Effects are unpredictable, maternal reflex tachycardia, may not alter fetal outcome

Always start with the lowest recommended doses; doses are the same as for nonpregnant patients.

to that observed with methyldopa and neonatal loss occurs at a similar rate as well. In one study, 47 neonates were studied 7 days after delivery from mothers treated with clonidine in doses ranging from 0.15 to 1.2 mg/day. No clinically significant hypotension or rebound hypertension was observed. Long-term follow-up of these children has not yet been reported.

B. Alpha-1 and Beta-adrenergic Blocking Agents

The alpha-1 blocker prazosin has been studied in a few small groups of patients with severe pregnancy-induced hypertension, often in combination with a beta-blocker. The uncontrolled reports that have been published suggest that prazosin can be effective, may aid in the avoidance of parenteral drugs, and thus far has not been associated with any adverse fetal effects.

Labetalol, which has multireceptor blocking properties (alpha-1, beta-blocking), has been studied extensively in pregnancy hypertension. It appears to have its greatest value in severe essential hypertension when it is administered either in the oral form or intravenously. The reported rate of BP control has been exceedingly high with labetalol, over 90%. Since the majority of studies with labetalol have been performed in women with severe hypertension, the rate of intrauterine growth retardation have been fairly high (25%). The high rate of growth retardation may be secondary to the hypertensive disease process since isotope studies have demonstrated that labetalol does not induce a reduction in uteroplacental blood flow.

Beta-blockers have also been widely used in pregnancy hypertension over the past decade. Earlier anecodotal reports of adverse side effects of neonatal bradycardia, depression, and hypoglycemia have not been supported as being common in clinical controlled trials with oral administration. However, there have been reports of delayed spontaneous respirations in the newborn following intravenous beta-blocker therapy in severely hypertensive women, occasionally even requiring temporary mechanical ventilation.

Many of the selective and nonselective agents have been evaluated in double-blind, placebo-controlled studies, including
acebutolol, atenolol, metoprolol, oxprenolol, propranolol, and
pindolol. In one study with atenolol in 120 women, doses of
100–200 mg daily lowered BP while standard bed rest and sodium
restriction had no effect. The beta-blocker therapy was associated
with a marked reduction in the incidence of severe hypertension
and the development of proteinuria. One-year follow-up of the
children in this study has shown no difference in growth indexes
or development despite the fact that a small incidence of neonatal
bradycardia was observed at birth.

Most of the beta-blockers have been studied in comparison to
alpha-methyldopa in pregnancy hypertension. Few differences in
efficacy have been noted; however, fewer maternal side effects occurred with the beta-blockers. Thus, many obstetricians have
begun to use beta-blockers regularly in their hypertensive pregnant
patients.

C. ACE Inhibitors and Calcium Channel Blockers

Compared to the adrenergic inhibitors, there is very limited information available on the benefits and side effects of the ACE
inhibitors and calcium channel blockers in the treatment of hypertension during pregnancy. There have been some anecodotal
reports with captopril and enalapril in the use of severe hypertension during pregnancy. These case reports have been mainly of
patients who did not achieve adequate control with other drugs,
or who had known renovascular hypertension. The ACE inhibitors
have usually been avoided because of the occurrence of increased
intrauterine death and stillbirth in pregnant animals (sheep, rab-
bits) treated with captopril. Development of renal failure in the
developing fetus has been reported in humans.

There have been a few studies with the dihydropyridine
calcium channel blockers, nifedipine and nitrendipine, in pregnancy hypertension. These reports have been confined to severe or
accelerated hypertension or short-term use in preeclampsia. While
the data show good maternal BP effects for short-term administra-

tion (< 6 weeks), it is not yet possible to give general recommendations on this class of drugs.

D. Diuretics

Hypertension during pregnancy, particularly PIH and preeclampsia, is associated with reduced plasma volume. Thus, the loop or thiazide diuretics are recommended only in cases of hypertension associated with congestive heart failure or other conditions of volume overload, such as renal failure. The potassium-sparing diuretic spironolactone has been reported to be effective in management of primary hyperaldosteronism during pregnancy but is not useful in the treatment of PIH.

E. Direct Vasodilators

Like methyldopa, hydralazine has been a commonly used drug for the treatment of moderate-to-severe hypertension during pregnancy for many years. Hydralazine has been shown to have no adverse effect on uterine blood flow as it lowers maternal BP. Despite its antihypertensive effects during pregnancy though, hydralazine has not been shown to have an impact on fetal outcome in mothers with moderate-to-severe hypertension. In combination with the beta-blockers pindolol, hydralazine was shown to delay the onset of preeclampsia until later in the third trimester.

VI. POSTPARTUM HYPERTENSION

It is often at this stage that the patient's primary physician is "invited" to participate in the management of the hypertension again. Most often, a chronically hypertensive patient in whom preeclampsia developed accompanied by accelerated hypertension prior to labor will return toward prepartum BP levels within a few days after delivery (as shown in the case presentation). At that time, the antihypertensive regimen that worked prior to the pregnancy can be resumed.

Ninety percent of patients who were normotensive prior to pregnancy and in whom PIH developed will become normotensive within a few weeks into the postpartum period. However, about 10% of these women will remain mildly hypertensive for several months and even up to 1 year postdelivery. These patients constitute a small group of individuals who have *postpartum hypertension*. Rarely, these women have postpartum thyroiditis and develop elevated heart rate and BP for a few weeks while their thyroid hormones are elevated, but these hemodynamic abnormalities clear up concomitant with the patient becoming euthyroid or hypothyroid. The cause of the majority of cases of postpartum hypertension remains an enigma. We have followed several women for a few years postdelivery and they have remained mildly hypertensive; all evaluations for secondary hypertension have been negative.

VII. MANAGEMENT OF HYPERTENSION
DURING LACTATION

During the last two decades, there has been an impressive upward trend in the number of women breast feeding. More than half of American mothers were breast feeding at the time of discharge from the hospital in a survey in the early 1980s; the figure may be even higher at the present time. We have followed many hypertensive mothers taking antihypertensive drugs and their infants while they were breast feeding for periods of up to 8 months. Many drugs can be prescribed for hypertensive, lactating women without any problems.

Drug transfer and concentration in breast milk are dependent on the physical and chemical properties of the drug. Most important are the degree of ionization, protein binding, molecular weight, and lipid solubility. The pH of human milk is about 7.0 while that of plasma is 7.4. Thus, antihypertensive drugs that are weak bases, such as the beta-blockers, are more like to transfer into the milk by ionization than weak acids, like methyldopa. Lipid-soluble drugs are also more likely to transfer into milk, since

Table 9.4   Antihypertensive Drug Excretion in Breast Milk

Drug	Daily dose (mg)	Average concentration in breast milk	Transfer to infant
Atenolol	100	0.6 μg/ml	10 μg/ml
Captopril	300	5.0 ng/ml	Not studied[a]
Chlorthalidone	50	0.4 μg/ml	Not studied
Clonidine	0.15	1.5 ng/ml	Not studied
Diltiazem	240	0.2 μg/ml	Not studied
Hydralazine	150	0.8 μg/ml	Not studied
Hydrochlorothiazide	50	0.12 μg/ml	<1 ng/ml
Methyldopa	1000	1.0 μg/ml	0.09 μg/ml
Metoprolol	200	1.7 μg/ml	Not studied
Nadolol	80	0.35 μg/ml	Not studied
Nitrendipine	20	5.0 ng/ml	Not studied[a]
Oxprenolol	160	0.13 μg/ml	Not studied
Propranolol	160	0.16 μg/ml	Not studied[a]
Timolol	15	16 ng/ml	Not studied
Verapamil	240	20 μg/ml	Not detected

[a]Anecodotally, no adverse effects on breast-fed infants found over short-term study.

such a high percentage of milk is fat. An estimate of the drug intake in an infant can be made if concentrations in breast milk and maternal dose are known. Of course, the relative dose to the infant must be adjusted for the small weight of a newborn in contrast to the adult for whom the drug was originally prescribed.

Table 9.4 shows the average concentrations of antihypertensive drugs in breast milk—not all agents have been studied, and there is almost no data on actual infant transfer (with measured samples in the plasma of the breast-fed infant). In general, the pharmacology of an antihypertensive drug in breast milk is much the same as it is in plasma, except that peak levels may be delayed in comparison (Fig. 9.2). Levels may linger in milk longer than in plasma as well, especially of drugs that are lipid soluble. If possible, we advise patients on once-daily antihypertensive drugs to avoid breast feeding at times of peak levels in plasma/milk.

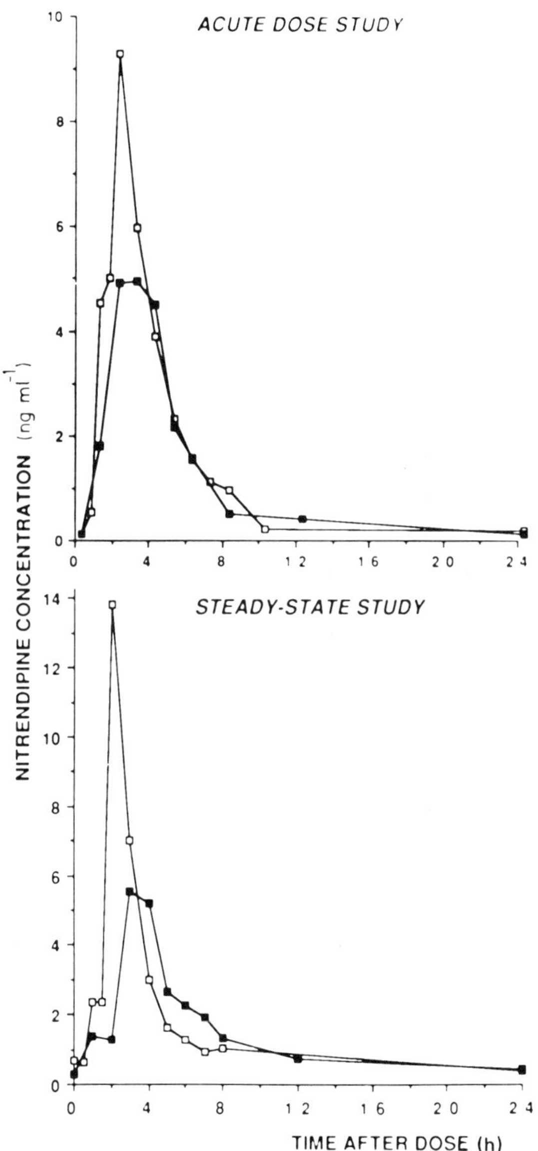

Figure 9.2 Profile of the antihypertensive drug nitrendipine in plasma (open squares) and breast milk (solid squares) from an acute dose and then after several days of administration. (From White WB, et al. *Eur J Clin Pharmacol* 1989; 36:531-534.)

Generally, both the physician and the breast-feeding mother have to weigh the risk/benefit ratio when the maternal medication is prescribed. Based on the data in Table 9.4, there are differences between the various antihypertensive agents in their ability to pass into the breast milk. Since most antihypertensive agents are excreted via breast milk, the obvious general recommendation would be to prescribe those agents found in minimal concentrations in the milk. Of course, the hemodynamic effects of an antihypertensive drug to an infant may theoretically occur even if the amount excreted in milk is extremely low; thus, evaluation of the infant by the pediatrician is necessary soon after therapy is begun.

Use of the diuretics as antihypertensive therapy should probably be avoided during lactation. Although excessive amounts do not appear in the milk (Table 9.4), they may suppress milk production. The beta-blockers do appear in breast milk, but numerous authors have commented that breast-fed infants do not appear to have any problems with the concentrations that do occur. The alpha-2 agonist methyldopa appears in the milk in lower concentrations than is found in maternal plasma. Our clinical experience with this agent in a few mothers demonstrated no long-term problems in their infants (follow-up is now over 5 years). Very few patients have been studied on the calcium channel blockers, but it is known that the level of the dihydropyridine nitrendipine is extremely low in the milk (Fig. 9.2). However, there is no clinical experience assessing the effect of this drug or any other calcium channel blocker on the breast-fed infant. Finally, the ACE inhibitor captopril is found in minuscule levels in the milk, actually only 0.01% of that found in maternal plasma. Thus, it is unlikely to have much of a hemodynamic effect on the breast-fed infant.

REFERENCES

Cockburn J, Moar VA, Ounsted N, et al. Final report on the study on hypertension during pregnancy: The effects of specific treatment on the growth and development of the children. *Lancet* 1982; 1:647–651.

Collins R, Yusuf S, Peto R. Overview of randomized trials of diuretics in pregnancy. *Br Med J* 1985; 290:17-19.

Liedholm H, Melander A. Drug selection in the treatment of pregnancy hypertension. *Acta Obstet Gynecol Scand* 1984; 118:49-60.

Redman C W G, Beillin L J, Bonnar J, et al. Fetal outcome in trial of antihypertensive treatment in pregnancy. *Lancet* 1976; 2:753-756.

Rubin P C. Treatment of hypertension in pregnancy. *Clin Obstet Gynecol* 1986; 13:307-326.

White W B. Management of hypertension during lactation. *Hypertension* 1984; 6:297-300.

White W B, Yeh S C, Krol G J. Nitrendipine in human plasma and breast milk. *Eur J Clin Pharmacol* 1989; 36:531-534.

With the advent of new and superior antihypertensive drugs, improved public awareness, and widespread high blood pressure (BP) screening programs, accelerated and emergency hypertension have become relatively rare. However, there are many clinical situations that one may not characterize as a well-known type of hypertensive emergency but in which parenteral drug therapy is obligatory. While the focus of this book has been on ambulatory medicine, those clinicians who practice hospital medicine will, on occasion, be involved in the management of hypertensive emergency. Thus, one major purpose of a chapter on this topic is to provide a forum for review of the parenteral antihypertensive drugs.

Classically, hypertensive emergency is defined as a life-threatening, acute elevation of the blood pressure that may occur with either essential or secondary forms of hypertension. There are no absolute BP values that constitute a diagnosis of hypertensive emergency. In most textbooks of medicine, markedly elevated diastolic BP values (over 130–140 mm Hg) and some overt signs of vascular injury (e.g., retinal hemorrhages) have been used to define the diagnosis. The presence of acute target organ injury, whether retinal, cardiac, renal, or neurological, is of much greater significance than the actual BP level itself. The following is a case illustration of a patient with a hypertensive emergency who presented with acute neurological signs.

I. ILLUSTRATIVE CASE

A 64-year-old man presented to the emergency room with the abrupt onset of diplopia, mild ataxia of gait, and marked elevation of the blood pressure to 250/150 mm Hg. He had a history of mild-to-moderate hypertension dating back nearly 35 years when he was inducted into the military. However, he never sought medical care following discharge from the service. Over the next three decades, he avoided physicians and his elevated BP went untreated.

On initial physical examination, the heart rate was 72 beats/min (bpm) and BP in both arms averaged 240–260/140–150 mm Hg on repeated determinations. Funduscopic examination demonstrated blurring of the nasal margin of both optic discs and venous congestion; no retinal hemorrhages or exudates were noted. Diplopia was confirmed since it disappeared when one eye was covered. The remainder of the neurological examination was normal. On cardiac examination, there was a regular rhythm interrupted by occasional premature beats (under 6 per minute) and a prominent 4th heart sound. There were no cardiac murmurs. Examination of the extremities showed mild ankle edema.

Urinalysis demonstrated + protein and was negative for glucose and ketones. Examination of the sediment showed occasional hyaline and granular casts; however, no red or white cells were seen. The serum creatinine was 1.9 mg/dl, blood urea nitrogen 28 mg/dl, and serum potassium 3.4 meq/l. The remaining blood chemistries and hematologic data were normal. Electrocardiogram showed a sinus rhythm with normal conduction times; there was a left-axis deviation of $-60°$ and voltage criteria for left ventricular hypertrophy. Furthermore, there were slightly inverted T waves in leads I, AVL, V4–V6 without depression of the ST segment. This finding could have been consistent with either lateral wall ischemia secondary to acute coronary insufficiency or a more chronic abnormality associated with the increased ventricular mass.

While the laboratory studies were being obtained, the staff in the emergency room prepared an intravenous solution of sodium nitroprusside diluted in 5% dextrose and protected it from light with a brown plastic bag around the bottle. The infusion was begun within approximately 15 min of arrival in the emergency room at an initial rate of 0.5 μg/kg/min. Blood pressure came down to only 230/110 mm Hg as the sodium nitroprusside was titrated up to 5 μg/kg/min by increases of 0.25–0.5 μg/kg/min at 10-min intervals. In addition, the heart rate increased to 90 bpm. The neurological symptoms persisted, and in fact, the patient developed dysarthria and drooping of the right nasolabial fold.

Since the BP response to the nitroprusside was incomplete and associated with a reflex tachycardia, a decision was made to add small doses of the intravenous alpha-beta blocker labetalol to the regimen. A slow intravenous injection of 10 mg labetalol was administered, followed by a constant infusion of the drug at 0.25 mg/min. Within about 10 min after the intravenous injection, the blood pressure was 180/90 mm Hg and heart rate fell to 80 bpm. The labetalol and nitroprusside infusions were continued at the stated doses over the next 12 hr in the intensive care unit. Myocardial infarction was ruled out with serial electrocardiograms and cardiac enzymes.

Computerized tomography of the brain on admission was normal. However, the morning after admission, the patient had developed a right hemiparesis; so the study was repeated and demonstrated a large infarction in the left parietooccipital region. The patient was kept at strict bed rest with his head flat, and special care was made to avoid upright posture. The nitroprusside was tapered off and labetalol continued parenterally at doses between

0.25 and 0.75 mg/min to maintain a systolic blood pressure between 160 and 200 mm Hg. The following day, the neurological symptoms appeared to be stable and oral labetalol was initiated at 200 mg every 12 hr. The intravenous labetalol was discontinued 1 hr after the first oral dose.

The hemiparesis and dysarthria persisted during the hospital course and blood pressure was fairly well controlled (150–160/90–100 mm Hg) on labetalol monotherapy. No attempt was made during hospitalization to lower BP further, and the labetalol was not increased so as to avoid potential postural hypotension. The patient was discharged to a rehabilitation facility.

II. CLINICAL CHARACTERISTICS OF HYPERTENSIVE EMERGENCY

Some of the entities that are associated with or cause hypertensive emergencies are listed in Table 10.1. The most specific clinical features of a hypertensive emergency include marked elevation of the BP and evidence of extensive target organ involvement. In the retina, findings include fresh, flame-shaped hemorrhages, exudates (which signify a resolving hemorrhage), and blurring of the disc margins secondary to papilledema. However, it is often difficult to differentiate the effects of diabetic versus hypertensive vascular disease in the retina. Not infrequently, a diabetic hypertensive with only modestly elevated BP will have retinal hemorrhages. An ophthalmology consultation should be requested as soon as possible to aid in diagnosis of a possible proliferative diabetic retinopathy which requires laser therapy.

A number of neurological symptoms are associated with accelerated or emergency hypertension—they range from headache and irritability to confusion, focal motor abnormalities, and visual disturbances. Unfortunately, some of the symptoms may be so mild that they are regarded as insignificant. At the other extreme, an encephalopathic state can develop which may present as seizures, stupor, or coma. Hypertensive encephalopathy carries a

Table 10.1   Clinical Entities Associated with Hypertensive Emergency

---

Cerebrovascular emergencies
  Intracranial hemorrhage
  Hypertensive encephalopathy
  Subarachnoid hemorrhage
  Acute thrombotic stroke
Cardiac emergencies
  Acute congestive heart failure
  Acute myocardial infarction or unstable angina pectoris
  Dissecting aortic aneurysm
  Postcoronary artery bypass or carotid bypass hypertension
Renal emergencies
  Acute renal failure—volume-dependent hypertension
  Renal artery thrombosis or injury
Pheochromocytoma
Rebound hypertension from sudden drug withdrawal
MAO inhibitor-tyramine interaction
Toxemia of pregnancy (discussed in Chapter 8)
Postoperative hypertension

---

grave prognosis and must be treated immediately with parenteral drug therapy.

Nonspecific signs and symptoms also occur with accelerated or emergent hypertension and include depression, fatigue, lethargy, nausea, and vomiting. In most textbooks, these symptoms are listed as possible findings with "malignant" hypertension, a term that suggests a poor outcome. The term is correct since if left untreated, severe hypertension with acute target organ injury has an exceedingly high mortality rate. To be more precise, however, malignant hypertension has always been associated with vascular wall damage secondary to fibrinoid necrosis. These vascular lesions occur in small vessel beds in the kidneys, brain, and mesenteric circulation and may be responsible, in part, for many of the nonspecific symptoms noted above.

A. Laboratory Analysis

If there is evidence on physical examination that some form of
vascular injury is in progress associated with markedly elevated BP,
it is unwise to wait for results of laboratory tests before initiating
therapy. However, since an intravenous line is required, blood and
urine samples can certainly be obtained prior to starting an antihypertensive agent. Laboratory studies may be especially important in the evaluation of secondary forms of hypertension
(Table 10.2). However, during the stress and/or discomfort of the
emergency room environment, plasma catecholamines or urinary
metanephrines may be elevated nonspecifically. If the level of
catecholamines is elevated, the results should be confirmed after
the BP is lowered and the patient is out of the critical care unit.

It also may be useful to perform a careful urinalysis to detect
renal involvement, as well the serum electrolytes, creatinine, and
blood urea nitrogen to evaluate the degree of renal dysfunction.
The level of renal function may be important in making decisions
about drug therapy. For example, it is known that cyanide
metabolites from sodium nitroprusside accumulate much more
rapidly in patients with moderate-to-severe renal insufficiency

Table 10.2 Useful Initial Laboratory Studies in Patients with Hypertensive Emergency

Study	Clinical utility/abnormalities
Complete blood count	Evaluation for small vessel damage associated with hemolysis
Renal function studies	Assessment of level of renal dysfunction may be important in drug selection
Catecholamine studies	Elevated in pheochromocytoma; however, acute MI, stroke, and pain can also elevate levels
Electrocardiography	Assess for presence of LVH, acute myocardial ischemia, evolving infarction, cardiac arrhythmias
Chest X-ray	Useful if symptoms of CHF present

MI, myocardial infarction; LVH, left ventricular hypertrophy; CHF, congestive heart failure.

than in those with normal renal function. A peripheral blood smear rules out the presence of microangiopathic hemolytic anemia (characterized by target cells and schistocytes) that is associated with fibrinoid necrosis of small arteries in patients with malignant hypertension.

In the emergency room, portable chest X-ray and electrocardiogram should be performed to assess whether there is any evidence of myocardial ischemia or congestive failure secondary to the elevated BP. If the presence of myocardial ischemia is established in the absence of pulmonary vascular congestion, an anti-adrenergic drug or ACE inhibitor may be superior to a direct vasodilator. If clinically relevant, computerized tomography of the head should be performed after the BP is lowered to a safer level (e.g., around 180/110 mm Hg).

III. RAPID BLOOD PRESSURE REDUCTION AND STROKE

In the majority of types of accelerated or emergent hypertension, BP can be lowered safely. In patients with neurological symptoms (e.g., the patient in the case at the beginning of this chapter), great caution must be taken. Rapid BP reduction is risky in a patient with either a cerebrovascular accident or a transient ischemic attack, or in an elderly patient with extensive cerebrovascular disease. While cerebral blood flow remains fairly constant in the nonischemic brain over a wide range of systemic arterial pressure, this autoregulation can be lost in the presence of cerebral injury. Thus, lowering BP too much or too rapidly can result in coma, seizures, or extension of cerebral injury.

Many neurologists at our institution feel that BP should not be lowered for the first 48–72 hr of an acute thrombotic stroke unless it is above 200/110 mm Hg. Furthermore, it is recommended that these patients have no abrupt postural changes that may result in transient cerebral hypotension. Potent vasodilators such as hydralazine and nifedipine should be avoided in stroke patients since they may transiently cause excessive hypotension and worsen cerebral ischemia. In patients with severely elevated BP, parenteral therapy should be used since it affords much tighter control and can be more rapidly reversed than an oral agent.

IV. DRUG THERAPY IN THE MANAGEMENT OF HYPERTENSIVE EMERGENCIES

A. Does the Patient Require Hospitalization?

Whether or not a patient is hospitalized for hypertension has become a complicated issue in recent years with all the major health policy changes that have occurred. In general, asymptomatic, severe hypertension that is not associated with clinical or laboratory evidence of acute target organ injury does not require acute hospitalization. A typical example of this situation is the patient who comes to an emergency room for an acute upper respiratory infection and is incidentally found to have a BP of 230/125 mm Hg. While it is worthwhile to assess the patient for retinal abnormalities and electrocardiographic changes, immediate outpatient follow-up (within 12–24 hr) by the patient's personal physician is reasonable.

Most physicians feel quite uncomfortable simply sending a patient home with diastolic BP over 130 mm Hg, even if he is entirely asymptomatic. I am one of those physicians, and there are two options: First, the simple laboratory tests mentioned above (Table 10.2) are obtained and a rapidly acting oral agent (Table 10.3) is administered. The patient is then observed for a reduction in BP in the office or emergency room over the next 2–3 hr and followed up the next day on the new medication. The second option is to admit the patient to the hospital for oral therapy and obtain the necessary studies for the evaluation of possible secondary hypertension. In patients who are unreliable (for whatever reason), option 2 is advisable.

B. Oral Agents

While most of the oral agents have been mentioned previously in this book, it has not been in the context of very severe hyperten-

Table 10.3 Oral Agents Recommended for Treatment of Very Severe, but Asymptomatic Hypertension

Agent	Dose	Onset of action	Side effects
Captopril	12.5-25 mg[a]	30-60 min	Excess hypotension
Clonidine	0.1 hourly for 5-6 hr	1-2 hr	Drowsiness, dry mouth, dizziness
Labetalol	100-200 mg[b]	1-2 hr	Postural hypotension, exacerbation of asthma
Minoxidil	2.5-5 mg	2 hr	Reflex tachycardia
Nifedipine	10 mg	15-30 min	Overshoot hypotension, reflex tachycardia

[a] In patients with congestive heart failure, initial dose = 6.25 mg.
[b] Use 100 mg in elderly patients.

sion. It is my personal bias that oral agents are not suitable for true hypertensive emergencies. While they may be easier to administer, their side effect potential is greater since there is less control and less ability to predict the effect on BP. However, they have a practical role in the therapy of asymptomatic, severely hypertensive patients.

1. ACE Inhibitors

Captopril is the only ACE inhibitor appropriate for use in this clinical situation because it has a rapid onset of action (30–60 min) and relatively short duration (peak effect over in 2 hr) compared to enalapril or lisinopril. Precipitous hypotension is a well-known side effect of captopril but is seen almost exclusively in patients with congestive heart failure (CHF) or those who have been quite volume-depleted from either gastroenteritis or diuretic therapy. In patients suspected of having a stimulated renin-angiotensin system from volume depletion or CHF, very small initial doses of 6.25-12.5 mg should be used. If the BP response is minimal after 1 hr, a second dose of 25 mg can be administered.

2. Alpha-2 Agonists

Clonidine has been used quite extensively in severe, urgent, and emergent hypertension. Because clonidine reduces systemic vascular resistance but causes no hemodynamically important increase in heart rate or cardiac output, it is safe to use in patients with ischemic heart disease and certainly is preferable to hydralazine or minoxidil. Most authors have suggested that clonidine be given in doses of 0.1–0.2 mg hourly for several hours until the BP is lowered to a satisfactory level. The success rate with the drug is high and excessive hypotension uncommon, but 5–6 hr is a fairly long time to wait for a safe BP level and the sedating side effects of clonidine may be problematic for some patients.

3. Alpha-Beta Blockers

Oral labetalol has a relatively rapid onset of action (about 1 hr) and has been studied fairly extensively in severe hypertension. It generally lowers BP significantly greater than a conventional alpha-1 blocker or non-ISA-containing beta-blocker. The more common side effects associated with labetalol relate to the alpha-blocking properties of the drug and include postural hypotension. The beta-blocking side effects of this drug are not pronounced, but labetalol is not the drug of choice in patients with bronchial asthma or poor left ventricular function.

4. Calcium Channel Blockers

The most extensively studied calcium channel blocker in severe hypertension and hypertensive emergency is nifedipine. The dihydropyridine calcium channel blockers (nicardipine, nifedipine, and nitrendipine) are all potent vasodilators, and nicardipine and nifedipine capsules have a rapid onset and short duration of action. The dihydropyridine calcium channel blockers are absorbed in the stomach and not by the sublingual or buccal mucosa. Thus, there is really no advantage to piercing the capsule and squirting the contents under the tongue! Two sophisticated pharmacological studies of nifedipine have demonstrated that the plasma concentration and pharmacodynamic effect was minimal while the drug was held in the oral cavity. Therefore, it is appropriate to ask patients to simply swallow the capsule.

In early clinical studies with nifedipine in very severe hypertension, there were almost no reports of side effects from its administration despite the fact that some patients experienced 80–100 mm Hg reductions in systolic BP within 20–30 min. Subsequently, reports appeared cautioning the use of nifedipine in severely hypertensive patients with known myocardial or cerebrovascular disease, since both extension of myocardial infarction and progression of stroke have been observed following excessive BP reduction with nifedipine administration.

5. Direct Vasodilators

I do not recommend the use of hydralazine or minoxidil as a first-line oral agent in severe hypertension. Both of these drugs markedly lower systemic vascular resistance and will likely impressively lower BP, but they may induce dramatic reflex sympathetic nervous system stimulation as well. In patients with known renal failure, minoxidil may be more successful than other agents in lowering BP. However, the drug should generally be used in combination with a loop diuretic and beta-adrenergic blocking drug.

C. Parenteral Agents

The parenteral agents recommended for hypertensive emergency are listed in Table 10.4. Older agents, such as reserpine and alpha-methyldopa, are considered to be obsolete since they offer no advantages over new drugs and have slower onsets of action and greater side effect profiles.

1. Diazoxide

We have not been using diazoxide for severe or accelerated hypertension in recent years at our hospital because we believe superior drugs have been developed. However, many physicians feel comfortable with this agent and continue to use it for hypertensive emergencies. Diazoxide reduces BP by direct vasodilation of

Table 10.4 Parenteral Agents Recommended for Hypertensive Emergency

Agent	Dose	Onset	Side effects
Diazoxide	25-100 mg bolus every 10 min	5 min	Precipitous hypotension
Enalaprilat	5-10 mg q4h	30-60 min	Excess hypotension
Hydralazine	10-20 mg i.v. over 5 min	10 min	Reflex tachycardia
Labetalol	5-20 mg slow i.v. followed by 0.25-2.0 mg/min	10-15 min	Bronchospasm in asthmatics
Nitroglycerin[a]	5-100 μg/min constant i.v.	10-15 min	Vasodilator headache, nausea
Phentolamine	5 mg i.v. bolus	5 min	Tachycardia
Sodium nitroprusside	0.5-10 μg/kg/min i.v.	5 min	Tachycardia, thiocyanate toxicity
Trimethaphan	1000 mg/liter (0.1%) i.v.	2-5 min	Hypotension, ileus, urinary retention

[a]Not recommended in the absence of myocardial ischemia.

arterioles and has little effect on capacitance vessels. Therefore, increases in heart rate and cardiac output will usually accompany the reduction in BP. When diazoxide was first introduced on the market, it was generally administered as a 300-mg bolus i.v. There was concern that if it was not given rapidly, serum protein binding would render the drug ineffective. Unfortunately, when i.v. bolus was given at this large dose, excessive hypotension was frequently encountered. When given in small injections of 25-50 mg or even by slow intravenous infusion (50 mg in 50 ml 5% dextrose over 30 min), the side effect of hypotension is reduced impressively. Contraindications to the use of diazoxide include suspicion of acute dissecting aneurysm or myocardial infarction. The reflex sympathetic stimulation may increase shearing force on the aortic tear and will likely increase myocardial oxygen demand.

2. Enalaprilat

Enalaprilat is the active metabolite of the ACE inhibitor enalapril and has been available for use as an intravenous antihypertensive agent for approximately 2 years. It lowers systemic vascular resistance and has little effect on cardiac output or heart rate (unless left ventricular function is depressed, and then cardiac output will improve secondary to improved stroke volume). In studies of severe or emergent hypertension, enalaprilat lowers BP within 10 min when given as an infusion of 5–10 mg over 20–30 min. This is then continued at 4–6 hr intervals. The major advantage of enalaprilat is in patients with severe hypertension and congestive heart failure.

3. Hydralazine

Like diazoxide, this direct vasodilator has also been abandoned by the medical service at our institution, but the drug continues to have regular use in pre- and postpartum hypertension (see Chapter 9). Unfortunately, the predictability of hydralazine in hypertensive emergencies is inconsistent. Thus, I cannot recommend it as a first-line agent in accelerated or emergent hypertension.

4. Labetalol

This alpha-beta blocking agent reduces BP through its lowering of systemic vascular resistance (the alpha-1 blocking effect). With intravenous injection or constant infusion, cardiac output is not altered while heart rate will be lowered modestly. When sympathetic tone is high and if heart rate is elevated (>80 bpm), labetalol will generally result in a larger reduction in heart rate. This drug can be administered either as a slow intravenous injection or by constant infusion. If the former method is chosen, an initial dose of 10–20 mg should be given over 3–5 min, and the result assessed in 10 min. If the effect on BP is quite small, a subsequent dose of 20–40 mg should be administered. This may be repeated up to a total of 300 mg over the course of 2 hr. Failure to achieve goal BP occurs in about 15% of patients with hypertensive emergency, especially if they have recently been taking anti-adrenergic drugs.

We prefer to use this drug as a constant infusion; generally it is administered as an intravenous injection of 10–20 mg, immediately followed by a constant infusion of 0.25 mg/min. This may be increased at 10–15-min intervals by 0.25 mg/min, depending on the goal BP. We have not observed much additional BP lowering effect following doses of 1.5–2.0 mg/min. In patients with hepatic and/or renal failure, dosage requirements may be less since labetalol is excreted by both organs. We have found labetalol to be particularly effective following major vascular procedures; others have reported its usefulness in severe hypertension associated with pheochromocytoma.

5. Nitroglycerin

Intravenous nitroglycerin is not a predictable antihypertensive agent; it may lower BP moderately through venodilation and reduction in preload to the heart. However, nitroglycerin may be very effective in lowering BP in patients with myocardial ischemia and angina pectoris at rest. This drug has been used as an anti-hypertensive successfully in patients whose BP rises significantly before, during, and following coronary artery surgery, while simultaneously having favorable effects on myocardial blood flow. Intravenous nitroglycerin can be used in combination with sodium nitroprusside in patients with acute myocardial infarction and severe hypertension.

6. Phentolamine

This is a very specific alpha-blocker used for hypertension associated with high circulating levels of catecholamines such as that seen in pheochromocytoma or in monoamine oxidase inhibitor-tyramine interaction. The use of phentolamine has decreased markedly since there are other less provocative tests for the diagnosis of pheochromocytoma and because intravenous labetalol or sodium nitroprusside can be used for the acute hypertension associated with pheochromocytoma.

7. Sodium Nitroprusside

This direct-acting and potent venodilating and arteriolar dilating drug has been one of the best agents available for hypertensive emergencies since it is fairly predictable and quite reliable. Its short half-life aids in rapid titration of the drug. An additional benefit of sodium nitroprusside is the improvement in left ventricular function that may occur in the failing heart secondary to a balanced reduction of preload and afterload.

One major drawback associated with the use of sodium nitroprusside is that the very potency that gives it utility has often led to restrictions on its use. These restrictions include invasive monitoring requirements or use in an intensive care unit setting. A skilled nurse must be following BP very closely while the patient is receiving the nitroprusside. We have had the opportunity to study patients receiving sodium nitroprusside and have found that on occasion, even slight increases in dose ($0.25\ \mu g/kg/min$) can markedly lower BP and result in symptomatic hypotension. Another concern frequently raised about sodium nitroprusside is thiocyanate toxicity following prolonged use. This appears to occur quite rarely and is almost unheard of unless the infusion is for more than 3 days or the patient has very poor renal function and is severely oliguric.

In a recent study we compared sodium nitroprusside to a new parenteral antihypertensive agent, fenoldopam, to evaluate effects on renal function in patients with severe hypertension. Fenoldopam is in a new class of drugs known as dopaminergic agonists; like dopamine, these drugs reduce renal vascular resistance and improve renal blood flow and sodium and water excretion. In this study (Fig. 10.1), fenoldopam resulted in a marked natriuriesis and diuresis while sodium nitroprusside had no effect on renal function but led to a significant retention of volume. These data have been supported by other studies in the past—thus, in patients with mild congestive failure or those whose BP does not respond well to sodium nitroprusside monotherapy, a loop diuretic should be used intermittently to avoid expansion of intravascular volume.

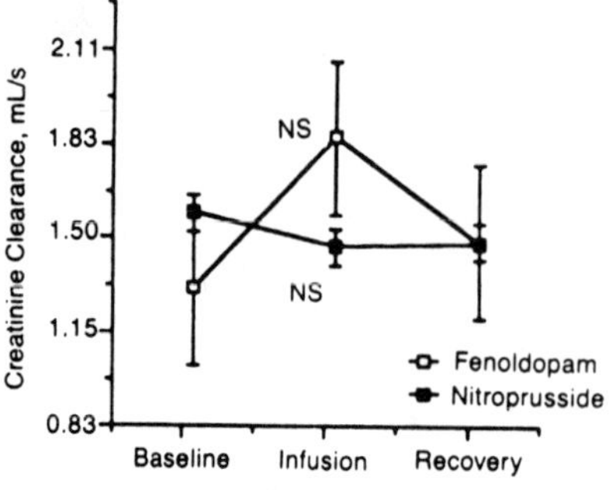

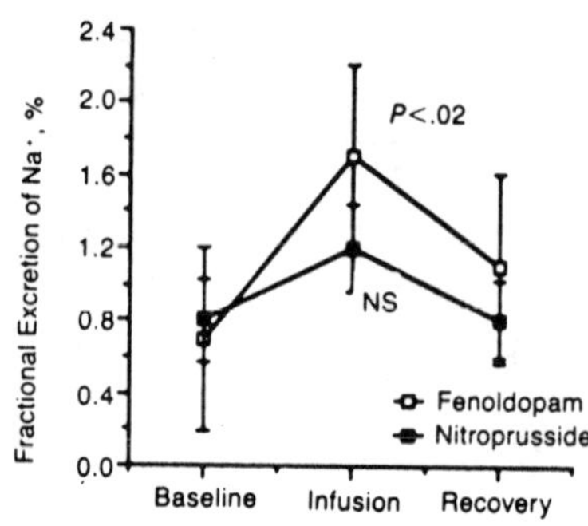

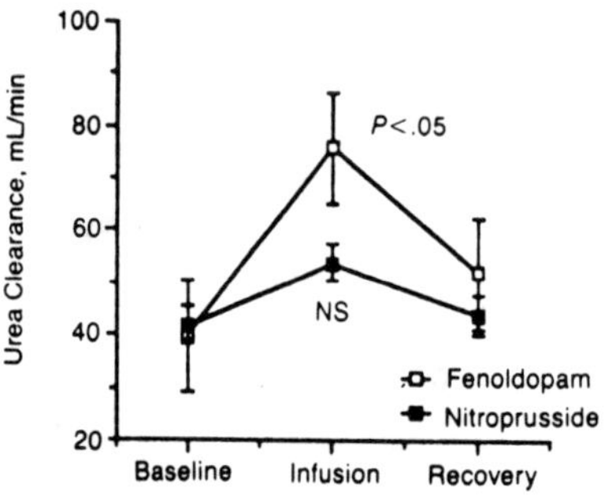

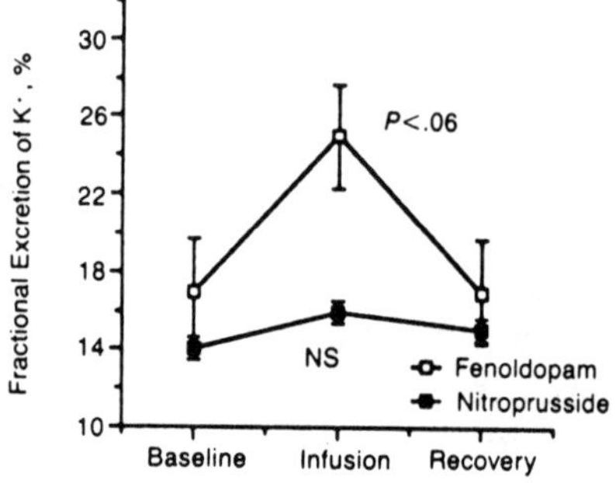

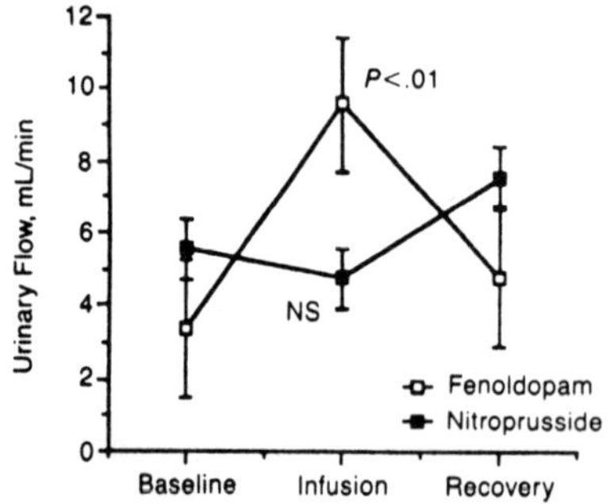

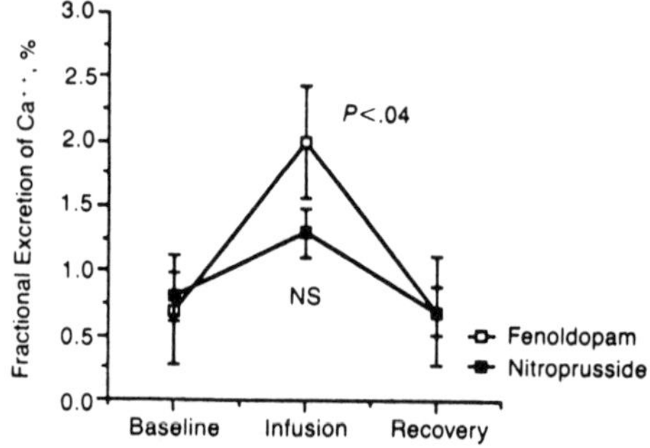

Figure 10.1 Various renal parameters following intravenous infusion of fenoldopam and sodium nitroprusside in patients with severe hypertension. (From White WB, Halley SE, *Arch Intern Med* 1989;149:870–874, with permission.)

8. Trimethaphan

This is an infrequently used agent because ganglionic blocking drugs that interrupt adrenergic control of vascular smooth muscle tone also have a similar effect in the gastrointestinal and genitourinary tract. Thus, some of the well-known side effects of this drug include paralytic ileus, urinary retention, severe postural hypotension, and bradycardia. However, many anesthesiologists prefer to use trimethaphan in the management of aortic dissection since it reduces cardiac output and aortic shearing force. Alternative therapy for aortic dissection includes concomitant administration of sodium nitroprusside and beta-adrenergic blockers.

Table 10.5 Preferred Drug Regimens in Various Types of Hypertensive Emergency Syndromes

Clinical syndrome	Preferred agent(s)	Agents to avoid
Acute myocardial infarction	Nitroprusside, nitroglycerin, labetalol	Diazoxide, hydralazine
Acute CHF	Nitroprusside, enalaprilat	Same as above
Aortic aneurysm (dissecting)	Nitroprusside + beta-blocker trimethaphan	Same as above
Adrenergic excess	Labetalol, phentolamine	
Encephalopathy	Nitroprusside, labetalol, diazoxide	Clonidine, methyldopa
Intracranial hemorrhage	Same as above	Same as above
Postoperative hypertension	Nitroprusside, labetalol, transdermal clonidine[a]	
Renal insufficiency	Labetalol, furosemide, nitroprusside	Enalaprilat[b]
Thrombotic stroke	Nitroprusside	Labetalol, clonidine, methyldopa

[a]Transdermal clonidine is useful as a short-term (not acute) postoperative therapy useful in patients with prolonged ileus who cannot take oral medications.
[b]Enalaprilat is contraindicated if bilateral renal artery stenosis is present.

V. COMMENTARY

As a long-time consultant to the intensive care unit on the management of severe hypertension in both medical and surgical patients, I have developed some bias regarding therapy for the different kinds of patients encountered who have hypertensive emergencies (Table 10.5). Some of the drugs mentioned in Table 10.4 no longer have an active role in the management of hypertensive emergency in our institution, but certainly they may be used successfully in other hospitals. The ideal parenteral antihypertensive agent has not been developed yet, but the agents that have become available in the past 5 years have proven to be major improvements over drugs that we were using just 15 years ago.

REFERENCES

Cohn J N, Burke L P. Nitroprusside. *Ann Intern Med* 1987;91:752–757.

Cressman M D, Vidt D G, Gifford R W, et al. Intravenous labetalol in the management of severe hypertension and hypertensive emergencies. *Am Heart J* 1984;107:980–985.

Ferguson R K, Vlasses P H. Hypertensive emergencies and urgencies. *JAMA* 1986;255:1607–1613.

Houston M C. Treatment of hypertensive emergencies and urgencies with oral clonidine loading and titration. *Arch Intern Med* 1986;146:586–589.

Luce B R, Ellrodt A G, Cameron J M, Riedinger M. Managing acute hypertension: cost considerations. *Am J Emerg Med* 1985;3:31–34.

White W B, Halley S E. Comparative renal effects of intravenous administration of fenoldopam mesylate and sodium nitroprusside in patients with severe hypertension. *Arch Intern Med* 1989;149:870–874.

Appendix

A Guide to the Use of Specific Antihypertensive Agents in Patients with Hypertension

This appendix is meant to complement the information on the antihypertensive drugs already discussed in the various chapters. Doses and dosing information follow the guidelines found in the manufacturer's package inserts and, to the best of the author's knowledge, are correct for use in clinical practice. The benefits and side effects given are those most commonly seen and are not to be considered exhaustive.

ALPHA-1 ADRENERGIC INHIBITORS

Mechanism of antihypertensive action: Inhibition of the action of catecholamines at the peripheral nerve terminal, specifically at alpha-1 receptor sites in the peripheral nervous system. Reduce systemic vascular resistance and systemic arterial pressure with no major effects on heart rate or cardiac output.

Alpha-1 Adrenergic Inhibitors (Continued)

Name: generic (trade)	Initial dose/dose interval (tablet or capsule sizes)	Maximally recommended dose in hypertension	First-choice agent or particular benefits	Common side effects/cautions
Prazosin (Minipress)	1 mg at bedtime, then bid (1, 2, and 5 mg capsules)	10 mg bid	Diabetics, chronic lung disease, hyperlipidemia	Postural hypotension, syncope
Terazosin (Hytrin)	1 mg at bedtime, then qd (1, 2, 5, and 10 mg tablets)	10 mg qd	Same as prazosin	Prolonged hypotension, con-fusion

bid, Twice daily; qd, once daily.

ALPHA-2 AGONISTS

Mechanism of antihypertensive action: Inhibition of release of catecholamine hormones from pre-synaptic nerve terminals located in the central nervous system. This induces a reduction in systemic vascular resistance with no major effect on cardiac output. The heart rate is generally unchanged or slightly reduced.

Name: generic (trade)	Initial dose/dose interval (tablet or capsule sizes)	Maximally recommended doses in hypertension	First-choice agent or particular benefits	Common side effects/cautions
Alpha-Methyldopa (Aldomet)	125–250 mg bid (125, 250, 500 mg tablets)	500 mg qid (or 750 mg bid)	None	Fatigue, sexual dysfunction
Clonidine (Catapres)	0.1 mg bid (or 0.2 mg qhs) (0.1, 0.2, 0.3 mg tablets)	1.2 mg bid	Diabetics, chronic lung diseases	Fatigue, dry mouth
Transdermal delivery (TTS)	0.1 mg/day/delivery (0.1, 0.2, 0.3 mg/day delivery systems)	0.3 mg/day/delivery	Same as tablets and patients who malabsorb	Contact dermatitis

| Guanabenz (Wytensin) | 4 mg bid (4, 8 mg tablets) | 12–16 mg bid | Diabetics, chronic lung diseases | Fatigue, confusion, dry mouth |
| Guanfacine (Tenex) | 1 mg at bedtime | 3 mg daily (bedtime) | None | Dry mouth, somnolence, weakness |

ANGIOTENSIN CONVERTING ENZYME INHIBITORS

Mechanism of antihypertensive action: Blocks the action of converting enzyme reducing circulating levels of the vasoconstrictor angiotensin II. A minor action of some agents in this class may also be to increase circulating levels of prostaglandins and kinins that have vasodilatory properties. In hypertension, these drugs lower systemic vascular resistance with little or no effect on cardiac output. Heart rate is either unchanged or slightly reduced.

Name: generic (trade)	Initial dose/dose interval (tablet or capsule sizes)	Maximally recommended doses in hypertension	First-choice agent or particular benefits	Common side effects/cautions
Captopril (Capoten)	12.5–25 mg qd or bid[a] (12.5, 25, and 50 mg tablets)	50 mg bid	Diabetes, congestive heart failure, chronic lung diseases, hyperlipidemia	Rash, dry cough, taste dysfunction; may worsen renal function in certain patients[b]
Enalapril (Vasotec)	2.5–5 mg qd or bid[a] (5, 10, and 20 mg tablets)	20 mg bid	Same as captopril	Same as captopril, angioedema is rare
Lisinopril (Prinivil, Zestril)	5–10 mg qd	40 mg qd	Same as captopril/enalapril	Same as captopril/enalapril

[a]Clinical experience and clinical trials suggest that captopril and enalapril should be given twice daily in patients with moderate to severe hypertension, while they may be adequate in once-daily dosing in the majority of mild hypertensives (diastolic BP > 90 Hg and < 104 mm Hg).
[b]Use lower doses in the elderly, patients taking diuretics, patients with congestive heart failure, diabetic patients with orthostatic hypertension, and patients with creatinine clearance rates < 30 ml/min.

BETA-ADRENERGIC BLOCKING AGENTS

Mechanism of antihypertensive action: A number of mechanisms have been proposed, including competitive inhibition of catecholamine hormones at vascular smooth muscles/synaptic junctions, blockade of release of presynaptic norepinephrine, and negative inotropic effects (myocardial). The net hemodynamic results include a reduction in cardiac output, heart rate, and blood pressure, and a small rise in systemic vascular resistance. The beta-blockers that contain intrinsic sympathomimetic activity (ISA) do not lower cardiac output at rest and reduce systemic vascular resistance.

Nonselective Agents (Block Both Beta-1 and Beta-2 Receptors)

Name: generic (trade)	Initial dose/dose interval (tablet or capsule sizes)	Maximally recommended doses in hypertension	First choice agent or particular benefits	Common side effects/cautions
Labetalol[a] (Normodyne, Trandate)	100 mg bid (100, 200, 300 mg tablets)	600 mg bid	Angina, peripheral vascular disease	Bronchospasm, postural hypotension, fatigue, ejaculatory failure
Nadolol (Corgard)	40 mg qd (40, 80, 120 mg tablets)	240 mg qd	Coronary heart disease, angina	Bronchospasm, fatigue, sexual dysfunction, claudication, left ventricular dysfunction rarely
Penbutolol[b] (Levatol)	10 mg qd (20 mg tablets)	40 mg qd	Coronary heart disease	Same as nadolol, less likely to induce claudication
Pindolol[b] (Visken)	5 mg bid (5, 10 mg tablets)	20 mg bid	Peripheral vascular disease, hyperlipidemia	Same as nadolol, but claudication less likely to occur secondary to ISA

| Propranolol (Inderal) | 40 mg bid (10, 20, 40, 60, 80 tablets) (LA, 40, 60, 80, 120 mg capsules) | 240 mg bid 240 mg qd for LA form | Coronary heart disease, post-MI | Similar to nadolol; nightmares reported |
| Timolol (Blocadren) | 2.5 mg bid (5, 10 mg tablets) | 20 mg bid | Coronary heart disease, post-MI | Same as propranolol and nadolol |

[a] Labetalol contains alpha-1 aderenergic blocking properties.
[b] Contains ISA.

Selective Agents (Block Predominantly the Beta-1 Receptor at Moderate Doses)

Name: generic (trade)	Initial dose/dose interval (tablet or capsule sizes)	Maximally recommended dose in hypertension	First-choice agent or particular benefits	Common side effects/cautions
Acebutolol[a] (Sectral)	200–400 mg qd (200 and 400 mg capsules)	800 mg qd or 600 mg bid	Coronary heart disease, angina, arrhythmias	Same as pindolol
Atenolol (Tenormin)	500 mg qd (50 and 100 mg tablets)	150 mg qd	Angina pectoris	Similar to nadolol, less bronchospasm
Metoprolol (Lopressor)	50 mg bid or qd (50 and 100 mg tablets)	200 mg bid	Coronary heart disease and post-MI	Similar to atenolol

[a] Acebutolol contains ISA.
post-MI, Following acute myocardial infarction.

CALCIUM CHANNEL BLOCKERS

Mechanism of antihypertensive action: Inhibition of calcium ion influx during depolarization of vascular smooth muscle which leads to dilatation of the smooth muscle. The major hemodynamic effect is reduction in systemic vascular resistance and arterial pressure. In general, the longer-acting calcium channel blockers have less vasodilatory-type side effects than the shorter-acting agents.

Name: generic (trade)	Initial dose/dose interval (tablet or capsule sizes)	Maximally recommended dose in hypertension	First-choice agent or particular benefits	Common side effects/cautions
Diltiazem (Cardiazem)	60 mg bid (30, 60, 90, 120 mg tablets) SR-form, 60, 90, 120 mg tablets)	180 mg bid 180 mg bid for SR form	Coronary heart disease, angina, uncomplicated post-MI	Peripheral edema, headache, bradycardia
Nicardipine (Cardene)	30 mg tid (30 mg capsules)	90 mg tid	Coronary heart disease, peripheral vascular disease	Peripheral edema, headache, flushing
Nifedipine (Procardia)	10 mg tid (10, 20 mg capsules) GITS-form (30, 60, 90 mg tablets)	40 mg tid 180 mg qd for GITS form	Coronary heart disease, angina coronary artery vasospasm, peripheral vascular disease	Peripheral edema, flushing, headache, precipitious hypotension
Nitrendipine (Baypress)	5 mg bid (5, 10, 20 mg tablets)	40 mg bid	Coronary heart disease, angina, peripheral vascular disease	Peripheral edema, flushing, headache
Verapamil (Calan, Isoptin)	40 mg bid (40, 80, 120 mg tablets) SR-form, 240 mg tablets	240 mg bid 480 mg qd for SR form	Cardiac arrhymias, coronary heart disease, systolic hypertension	Bradycardia, constipation

SR, sustained release; GITS, gastrointestinal transport system; MI, myocardial infarction.

DIURETICS

Mechanism of antihypertensive action: There are two possible mechanisms elucidated for the hypotensive effect of the various classes of diuretics. The likely short-term effect is secondary to increased renal excretion of sodium and water and reduction of plasma volume and cardiac output. However, the more long-term antihypertensive effects of diuretics are secondary to a reduction in systemic vascular resistance (the etiology of reduced vascular resistance is unknown).

Name: generic (trade)	Initial dose/dose interval (tablet or capsule sizes)	Maximally recommended dose in hypertension	First-choice agent or particular benefits	Common side effects/cautions
Saluretic-antihypertensive[a]				
Indapamide (Lozol)	2.5 mg qd (2.5 mg tablets)	5 mg qd	Edema, CHF	Hypokalemia, hyperuricemia (less so than thiazides)
Metolazone (Zaroxylyn, Diulo)	2.5 mg qod (2.5, 5, 10 mg tablets)	10 mg qd	Renal failure, severe edema, CHF	Severe metabolic disturbances (hypokalemia, hyponatremia, hypochloremia)
Loop Diuretics[a]				
Bumetanide (Bumex)	0.5 mg qd (0.5, 1, 2 mg tablets)	5 mg qd	CHF, edema, renal insufficiency	Volume depletion, electrolyte disturbances
Furosemide (Lasix)	20 mg bid (20, 40, 80 mg tablets)	80 mg bid (higher in *CRF*)	Same as bumetanide	Same as bumetanide
Potassium-sparing diuretics[a]				
Amiloride (Midamor)	5 mg qd (with thiazide) (5 mg tablets)	10 mg bid	Hypokalemia 2° kaliuretic diuretics	Hyperkalemia (esp. in diabetics, renal insufficiency patients)
Spironlactone (Aldactone)	25 mg bid (25, 50, 100 mg tablets	100 mg bid	Cirrhosis and volume overload; hypokalemia	Same as amiloride
Triameterene (Dyrenium)	50 mg bid	100 mg bid	Same as above	Same as above; renal calculi

Diuretics (Continued)

Thiazide and thiazide-like diuretics

Bendroflu-methiazide (Naturetin)	2.5 mg qd (5, 10 mg tablets)	10 mg qd	Systolic hypertension, peripheral edema	Electrolyte disturbances: hypokalemia and natremia, hyperuricemia, elevates total cholesterol
Benzathiazide (Exna)	25 mg qd (50 mg tablets)	100 mg qd	Same as above	Same as above
Chlorthalidone (Hygroton, Thalitone)	25 mg qd (25, 50, 100 mg tablets)	50 mg qd	Same as above	Same as above but hypokalemia may be more severe
Chlorthiazide (Diuril)	250 mg qd (250, 500 mg tablets)	1000 mg qd	Same as above	Same as bendroflumethiazide
Hydrochlorthiazide (Esidrix, Hydrodiuril, Oretic)	12.5–25 mg qd (25, 50, 100 mg tablets)	50 mg qd	Same as above	Same as above
Hydroflumethiazide (Saluron)	25 mg qd (50 mg tablets)	100 mg qd	Same as above	Same as above
Methyclothiazide (Enduron)	2.5 mg qd (2.5, 5 mg tablets)	5 mg qd	Same as above	Same as above
Polythiazide (Renese)	1 mg qd (1, 2, 4 mg tablets)	4 mg qd	Same as above	Same as above
Trichlormethiazide (Naqua)	1 mg qd (2, 4 mg tablets)	4 mg qd	Same as above	Same as above

[a]These agents are not considered first-line diuretics in the management of hypertension; the loop diuretics and saluretics should only be used in the presence of refractory edema or significant renal impairment (creatinine clearance < 20 ml/min).
All diuretics also have the potential to induce excessive volume contraction and, in patients with renal insufficiency, worsened azotemia.
CHF, Congestive heart failure. CRF, chronic renal failure.

PERIPHERAL VASODILATORS

Mechanism of antihypertensive action: The precise mechanism of the directly acting vasodilators is unknown. Some studies suggest that calcium ion transport is altered in vascular smooth muscle reducing contractility. The hemodynamic effects of these agents is a marked reduction in systemic vascular resistance, often associated with a sympathetically mediated rise in heart rate and cardiac output (if used in the absence of an adrenergic inhibitor). These drugs are neither initial therapy for hypertension nor should they be used without an adrenergic-blocking drug.

Name: generic (trade)	Initial dose/dose interval (tablet or capsule sizes)	Maximally recommended dose in hypertension	Particular benefits	Common side effects/cautions
Hydralazine (Apresoline)	25 mg bid (25, 50, 100 mg tablets)	100 mg bid	None	Flushing, palpitations, tachycardia
Minoxidil[a] (Loniten)	5 mg qd or 2.5 mg bid (2.5, 10 mg tablets)	40 mg bid	Useful in refractory hypertension associated with renal failure	Volume retention, CHF, tachycardia

[a]Minoxidil should always be prescribed in conjunction with a loop diuretic and beta-adrenergic blocking drug.

MISCELLANEOUS AGENTS THAT ARE OLDER BUT STILL IN USE

Name: generic (trade)	Initial dose/dose interval (tablet or capsule sizes)	Maximally recommended dose in hypertension	Particular benefits	Common side effects/cautions
Guanethidine (Ismelin)	10 mg qd (10, 25 mg tablets)	50 mg qd	None	Syncope/postural hypotension, retrograde ejaculation, diarrhea

Miscellaneous Agents That are Older but Still in Use (Continued)

| Phenoxyben-
zamine
(Dibenzy-
line) | 10 mg bid (10 mg
capsules) | 40–60 mg tid | Pheochromocytoma | Postural hypotension, inhibition
of ejaculation, nasal conges-
tion |
| Reserpine
(generic) | 0.125 qd or qod (0.125,
0.25 mg tablets) | 0.5 mg qd | None other than low cost | Sedation, depression, nasal
stuffiness |

DIURETICS IN COMBINATION WITH OTHER ANTIHYPERTENSIVE DRUGS

There are many antihypertensive drugs that have been combined with a diuretic in the same tablet for the patient's convenience and to improve compliance. One problem with combination drugs is evaluating adverse side effects in a given individual. We have never used combination antihypertensive drugs as initial therapy with the exception of some of the potassium-sparing diuretics. However, if an individual has been taking an antihypertensive agent along with a small dose of diuretic, is well-controlled, and the exact combination exists in one tablet, then substituting the combination drug could improve compliance and cost less. Listed below are some of the more commonly used combination drugs.

Name	Antihypertensive drug, dose	Diuretic, dose	Usual dosing interval
Aldochlor, 150 or 250	Alpha-methyldopa, 250 mg	Chlorthiazide, 150, 250 mg	bid
Aldoril, 15, 25, D30, D50	Alpha-methyldopa, 250 or 500 mg	Hydrochlorthiazide, 15, 25, 30, 50 mg	bid
Apresazide, 25/50, 50/50, and 50/100	Hydralazine, 25, 50, 100 mg	Hydrochlorothiazide, 25, 50, 50 mg	bid
Capozide, 25/15, 25/25, 50/15, and 50/25	Captopril, 25, 50 mg	Hydrochlorothiazide, 15, 25 mg	qd or bid

Combipres, 0.1, 0.2, 0.3	Clonidine, 0.1, 0.2, or 0.3 mg	Chlorthalidone, 15 mg	bid
Corzide, 40/5 and 80/5	Nadolol, 40 or 80 mg	Bendroflumethiazide, 5 mg	qd
Diupres-250 and 500	Reserpine, 0.125 mg	Chlorthiazide, 250, 500 mg	qd
Diutensin-R	Reserpine, 0.1 mg	Methyclothiazide, 2.5 mg	qd
Enduronyl (Forte)	Deserpindine, 0.25 and 0.5 mg	Methychlothiazide, 5 mg	qd
Esimil	Guanethidine, 10 mg	Hydrochlorothiazide, 25 mg	qd
Hydropres 25 and 50	Reserpine, 0.125 mg	Hydrochlorothiazide, 25, 50 mg	
Inderide, 40/25 and 80/25	Propranolol, 40 or 80 mg	Hydrochlorthiazide, 25 mg	bid
Inderide LA, 80/50, 120/50, or 160/50	Propranolol-LA, 80, 120, 160 mg	Hydrochlorothiazide, 50 mg	qd
Minizide, 1, 2, and 5	Prazosin, 1, 2, or 5 mg	Polythiazide, 0.5 mg	bid
Normozide, 100/25, 200/25, 300/25	Labetalol, 100, 200, or 300 mg	Hydrochlorothiazide, 25 mg	bid
Oreticyl, 25, 50, and Forte	Deserpidine, 0.125 or 0.25 mg	Hydrochlorothiazide, 25 or 50 mg	qd
Rauzide	Powdered rauwolfia, 50 mg	Bendroflumethiazide, 4 mg	qd
Salutensin (Demi)	Reserpine, 0.125 mg	Hydroflumethiazide, 25 or 50 mg	qd
Ser-Ap-Es	Reserpine, 0.1 mg, and Hydralazine, 25 mg	Hydrochlorothiazide, 15 mg	qd
Tenoretic 50, 100	Atenolol, 50 or 100 mg	Chlorthalidone, 25 mg	qd
Timolide	Timolol, 10 mg	Hydrochlorothiazide, 25 mg	bid
Vasoretic	Enalapril, 10 mg	Hydrochlorothiazide, 25 mg	qd

Index

R

S

About the Author

WILLIAM B. WHITE is Associate Professor of Medicine and Chief of the Section of Hypertension and Vascular Diseases, University of Connecticut School of Medicine, Farmington. The author or coauthor of over 90 publications, he is a Fellow of the American College of Physicians, and a member of the American Heart Association, American Society of Clinical Pharmacology, and International Society of Hypertension. Dr. White also serves on the editorial board of *Clinical Pharmacology and Therapeutics* and is a consultant to numerous hypertension, cardiology, and pharmacology journals. He received the B.S. degree from Emory University, Atlanta, Georgia and M.D. degree from the Medical College of Georgia, Augusta.